Interpreting Clinical Investigations in ICU

Interpreting Clinical Investigations in ICU

Editors

Rahul Anil Pandit
DA MD (Anesthesia) FJFICM FCICM (Australia) FCCP EDIC IFCCM
Chair
Department of Critical Care and Emergency Medicine
Sir HN Reliance Foundation Hospital
Mumbai, Maharashtra, India

Charudatt Vaity
MD (Medicine) DNB (Medicine) MRCP (UK) FFICM (UK) EDIC IFCCM
Additional Director
Department of Critical Care
Sir HN Reliance Foundation Hospital
Mumbai, Maharashtra, India

Bindu Mulakavalupil
DA DNB (Anesthesia) EDIC IDCCM
Chief Intensivist
Department of Liver and Transplant ICU
Sir HN Reliance Foundation Hospital
Mumbai, Maharashtra, India

Foreword
Shashank R Joshi

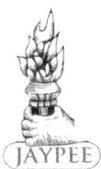

JAYPEE BROTHERS MEDICAL PUBLISHERS
The Health Sciences Publisher
New Delhi | London

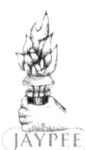 **Jaypee Brothers Medical Publishers (P) Ltd.**

Headquarters

Jaypee Brothers Medical Publishers (P) Ltd
EMCA House, 23/23-B
Ansari Road, Daryaganj
New Delhi 110 002, India
Landline: +91-11-23272143, +91-11-23272703
+91-11-23282021, +91-11-23245672
Email: jaypee@jaypeebrothers.com

Corporate Office

Jaypee Brothers Medical Publishers (P) Ltd
4838/24, Ansari Road, Daryaganj
New Delhi 110 002, India
Phone: +91-11-43574357
Fax: +91-11-43574314
Email: jaypee@jaypeebrothers.com

Overseas Office

JP Medical Ltd.
83, Victoria Street, London
SW1H 0HW (UK)
Phone: +44 20 3170 8910
Fax: +44 (0)20 3008 6180
Email: info@jpmedpub.com

Website: www.jaypeebrothers.com
Website: www.jaypeedigital.com

© 2024, Jaypee Brothers Medical Publishers

The views and opinions expressed in this book are solely those of the original contributor(s)/author(s) and do not necessarily represent those of editor(s) or publisher of the book.

All rights reserved. No part of this publication may be reproduced, stored or transmitted in any form or by any means, electronic, mechanical, photocopying, recording or otherwise, without the prior permission in writing of the publishers.

All brand names and product names used in this book are trade names, service marks, trademarks or registered trademarks of their respective owners. The publisher is not associated with any product or vendor mentioned in this book.

Medical knowledge and practice change constantly. This book is designed to provide accurate, authoritative information about the subject matter in question. However, readers are advised to check the most current information available on procedures included and check information from the manufacturer of each product to be administered, to verify the recommended dose, formula, method and duration of administration, adverse effects and contraindications. It is the responsibility of the practitioner to take all appropriate safety precautions. Neither the publisher nor the author(s)/editor(s) assume any liability for any injury and/or damage to persons or property arising from or related to use of material in this book.

This book is sold on the understanding that the publisher is not engaged in providing professional medical services. If such advice or services are required, the services of a competent medical professional should be sought.

Every effort has been made where necessary to contact holders of copyright to obtain permission to reproduce copyright material. If any have been inadvertently overlooked, the publisher will be pleased to make the necessary arrangements at the first opportunity.

Inquiries for bulk sales may be solicited at: jaypee@jaypeebrothers.com

Interpreting Clinical Investigations in ICU

First Edition: **2024**

ISBN: 978-93-5696-392-4

Contributors

Bindu Mulakavalupil
DA DNB (Anesthesia) EDIC IDCCM
Chief Intensivist
Department of Liver and Transplant ICU
Sir HN Reliance Foundation Hospital
Mumbai, Maharashtra, India

Charudatt Vaity
MD (Medicine) DNB (Medicine) MRCP (UK) FFICM (UK) EDIC IFCCM
Additional Director
Department of Critical Care
Sir HN Reliance Foundation Hospital
Mumbai, Maharashtra, India

Gagana BN
MD DrNB (Critical Care Medicine)
Senior Resident
Intensive Care Unit
Tata Memorial Hospital
Mumbai, Maharashtra, India

Gurudas Sadanand Pundpal
MD DNB (Pulmonary Medicine) FNB (Critical Care Medicine)
Consultant
Department of Intensivist and Pulmonologist
Wockhardt Hospital
Mumbai, Maharashtra, India

Hamza Dalal
MD (Medicine) DNB (Clinical Hematology)
Consultant
Department of Hematology
Fortis Hospital
Mumbai, Maharashtra, India

Haresh Dodeja
MD DNB MNAMS
Director Nephrology
Fortis Hospital Mulund
Mumbai, Maharashtra, India

Hozefa Runderawala
MBBS DNB (Medicine) DrNB (Gastro) ESEGH (MRCP-SCE, UK)
Consultant
Department of Gastroenterology
Saifee Hospital
Mumbai, Maharashtra, India

Jitendra Choudhary
MD FNB (Critical Care Medicine) IDCCM EDIC
Senior Consultant and Head
Department of Critical Care Medicine
Fortis Hiranandani Hospital, Vashi
New Mumbai, Maharashtra, India

Nachiket Desai
MD (Internal Medicine) Fellowship in Nephrology
Consultant
21st Century Hospital
Vapi, Gujarat, India

PragnaSree R
DNB (Anesthesia) IDCCM MD IDCCM (Critical Care Medicine)
Consultant
Department of Critical Care
Sir HN Reliance Foundation Hospital
Mumbai, Maharashtra, India

Pramila Chandan
MD DrNB (Critical Care Medicine)
Senior Resident
Intensive Care Unit
Tata Memorial Hospital
Mumbai, Maharashtra, India

Rahul Anil Pandit
DA MD (Anesthesia) FJFICM FCICM (Australia) FCCP EDIC IFCCM
Chair
Department of Critical Care and Emergency Medicine
Sir HN Reliance Foundation Hospital
Mumbai, Maharashtra, India

Foreword

It gives me great pleasure to present **"Interpreting Clinical Investigations in ICU"**. This book fills an important gap in critical care literature, being a comprehensive guide to requesting and interpreting a wide range of diagnostic tests. Dr Rahul Anil Pandit and team have collated a huge amount of information into a crisp volume. Its size, scope, and relevance means that it is likely to be used daily as a quick reference and aide-memoire. The fact that it is written by experienced clinicians, including trainees, is evident from its practical approach and focus on the patient. Its use will ensure that the right investigations are done first time, reducing unnecessary testing and enabling faster and more accurate diagnosis.

Shashank R Joshi
MD DM FRCP FACE FACP
Padma Shri Awardee
Consultant Endocrinologist
Lilavati and Sir HN Reliance Foundation Hospital, Joshi Clinic, Mumbai
Past President, Association of Physicians of India
Dean, Indian College of Physicians
Past President
Endocrine Society of India
Research Society for Study of Diabetes in India
Past Chair, International Diabetes Federation, Southeast Asia Region
Past President, International College of Nutrition

Preface

In the high-stress environment of the intensive care unit (ICU), healthcare professionals are faced with the critical task of interpreting clinical investigations to make life-saving decisions. This book serves as a comprehensive guide for clinicians, nurses, and students working in the ICU, providing essential knowledge and practical insights into the art and science of deciphering the myriad of diagnostic tests and assessments that are integral to patient care in this challenging setting.

This book has been meticulously crafted to bridge the gap between theory and practice, offering a clear and concise understanding of the most clinical investigations. It is our hope that by delving into the pages of the book, you will not only enhance your proficiency in interpreting clinical data but also gain a deeper appreciation for the crucial role these investigations play in delivering the best possible care to critically ill patients.

We have gathered a team of expert contributors, each bringing their unique perspectives and experiences from the front lines of critical care medicine. Through a combination of real-life case studies, evidence-based guidelines, and practical tips, this book will empower you to navigate the intricacies of interpreting clinical investigations with confidence.

As you embark on this journey through the world of clinical investigations in the ICU, remember that you are an integral part of a dedicated team working tirelessly to save lives. Your commitment to learning and improving your skills will undoubtedly have a profound impact on the patients under your care.

Thank you for choosing this book as your guide. We wish you success in your pursuit of excellence in the art of interpreting clinical investigations, and most importantly, in your mission to provide the highest standard of care to those who rely on your expertise.

Rahul Anil Pandit
Charudatt Vaity
Bindu Mulakavalupil

Acknowledgments

It has been a difficult but incredibly rewarding journey to write the book **"Interpreting Clinical Invsetigations in ICU"**, and we are grateful to many people for their assistance and encouragement along the way. We want to thank everyone who has helped with this job from the bottom of our heart. Above all, we sincerely thank the committed critical care specialists who work nonstop on the front lines, saving lives each and every day. We would want to express our gratitude to our mentors and colleagues in the critical care and allied specialties for their significant contributions. We would want to express our gratitude to the patients and their families who have so kindly allowed us to benefit from their experiences. We would like to express our special gratitude to Shri Jitendar P Vij (Group Chairman), Mr Ankit Vij (Managing Director), Mr Ms Mani (Group President), Ms Chetna Malhotra (Senior Director—Professional Publishing, Marketing, and Business Development), Ms Pooja Bhandari (Director—Production), Asmi Bharati (Development Editor) and the staff of M/s Jaypee Brothers Medical Publishers (P) Ltd, New Delhi, India.

Contents

Chapter 1. Acid–base Balance and Disorders and Stepwise Approach to their Interpretation with Case Scenario...........1
Jitendra Choudhary, Bindu Mulakavalupil, Rahul Anil Pandit
- Case Scenario 1: Acute Respiratory Alkalosis *4*
- Case Scenario 2: Chronic Respiratory Alkalosis *6*
- Case Scenario 3: Acute Respiratory Acidosis *7*
- Case Scenario 4: Chronic Respiratory Acidosis *7*
- Case Scenario 5: Metabolic Acidosis *7*
- Case Scenario 6: Lactic Acidosis *9*
- Case Scenario 7: Mixed Acidosis Hagma + Nagma *11*
- Case Scenario 8: Metabolic Alkalosis *12*

Chapter 2. Common Electrolyte Imbalances...........17
Pramila Chandan, PragnaSree R, Gagana BN, Charudatt Vaity
- Case Scenario 1: Pseudohyponatremia *17*
- Case Scenario 2: Hypoosmolar Hyponatremia *18*
- Case Scenario 3: Psychogenic Polydipsia *20*
- Case Scenario 4: Acute Tubular Necrosis *21*
- Case Scenario 5: Hyponatremia with Thiazides *22*
- Case Scenario 6: SIADH *23*
- Case Scenario 7: Hypernatremia *23*
- Case Scenario 8: Hypokalemia *25*
- Case Scenario 9: Hyperkalemia *27*
- Case Scenario 10: Hypocalcemia *29*
- Case Scenario 11: Hypercalcemia *31*
- Case Scenario 12: Hypophosphatemia *33*
- Case Scenario 13: Hyperphosphatemia *35*

Chapter 3. Case Scenarios and Interpretations of their Investigations...........37
Hamza Dalal, Nachiket Desai, Hozefa Runderawala, Haresh Dodeja, Bindu Mulakavalupil

- **3.1. Anemias**...........37
  - Case Scenario 1: Microcytic Anemia *37*
  - Case Scenario 2: Macrocytic Anemia *40*
  - Case Scenario 3: Normocytic Anemia *43*
  - Case Scenario 4: Pancytopenia *45*
  - Case Scenario 5: Microangiopathic Hemolytic Anemia *47*

- **3.2. Thrombocytopenia**...........51
  - Case Scenario *52*

- **3.3. Infection Markers and their Interpretation**...........55
  - Case Scenario *55*

3.4. Interpretation of Coagulation Studies 59
- Case Scenario 63

3.5. Renal Function Tests Urine Analysis 65
- Case Scenario 1: Azotemia 69
- Case Scenario 2: Nephrotic Syndrome 70
- Case Scenario 3: Renal Tubular Acidosis 71
- Case Scenario 4: Postobstructive Diuresis 73
- Case Scenario 5: Rhabdomyolysis 74

3.6. Liver Function Tests 77
- Case Scenario 1: Acute on Chronic Liver Failure 78
- Case Scenario 2: Cholestasis 80

3.7. Pancreatitis 81
- Case Scenario 81

3.8. Acute Coronary Syndrome 82
- Case Scenario 82

Chapter 4. Endocrinological Abnormalities 83
Gurudas Sadanand Pundpal, Rahul Anil Pandit
- Case Scenario 1: Adrenal Insufficiency 83
- Case Scenario 2: Conn's Syndrome 84
- Case Scenario 3: Hyperosmolar Hyperglycemic State 86
- Case Scenario 4: Diabetic Ketoacidosis 88
- Case Scenario 5: Hypoglycemia 92

Chapter 5. Toxicology 95
PragnaSree R, Charudatt Vaity
- Case Scenario 1: Pyroglutamic Acidosis 95
- Case Scenario 2: Lithium 97
- Case Scenario 3: Tricyclic Antidepressant Toxicity 99
- Case Scenario 4: Propofol Infusion Syndrome 101
- Case Scenario 5: Ethylene Glycol Poisoning 103
- Case Scenario 6: Methemoglobinemia 105
- Case Scenario 7: Cyanide Toxicity 107
- Case Scenario 8: Salicylate Toxicity 110
- Case Scenario 9: Acetaminophen Toxicity 111
- Case Scenario 10: Paraquet Poisoning 114
- Case Scenario 11: Aluminium Phosphide Poisoning 116
- Case Scenario 12: Organophosphorus Poisoning 118

Chapter 6. Artifacts 122
Pramila Chandan, Bindu Mulakavalupil
- Case Scenario 1: Diluted Blood Sample 122
- Case Scenario 2: EDTA Effect 123
- Case Scenario 3: Hemolyzed Sample 124

Index 127

CHAPTER 1

Acid–base Balance and Disorders and Stepwise Approach to their Interpretation with Case Scenario

Jitendra Choudhary, Bindu Mulakavalupil, Rahul Anil Pandit

INTRODUCTION

Arterial blood gases (ABGs) continue to be the established approach for diagnosing, classifying, and measuring respiratory and metabolic dysfunction. Systematic approaches to the diagnosis of acid–base disorders involve three critical steps.[1]

The first step is to have a comprehensive clinical evaluation that encompasses a detailed analysis of the patient's medical history, physical examination, and preliminary diagnostic tests. This analysis should facilitate a clinical determination regarding the probable acid–base problem and the potential differential diagnoses. Mixed disorders can present a challenge in terms of identification, as relying just on historical information and physical examination is typically inadequate for establishing a definitive diagnosis. The second step involves doing a methodical assessment of the ABG. The third step involves synthesizing all the available information and doing an analysis of the diagnosis.[2]

It is necessary to validate all ABGs by employing the equation $\{H^+\} = 24 \times PCO_2/HCO_3$.[3] Because of the near-linear relationship between pH and [H^+] in the pH interval of 7.25–7.5, an estimated [H^+] can be made by a "rule of 80" (subtracting the last two digits of the pH from 80 approximates [H^+]).

The present discourse aims to explicate the systematic interpretation rules utilized in the analysis of ABG results. Firstly, it is necessary to examine the oxygenation and afterward compute either the alveolar–arterial (A–a) gradient or the ratio of partial pressure of arterial oxygen (PaO_2) to fraction of inspired oxygen (FiO_2). Abnormally low levels of oxygen pose the greatest risk to one's life and are therefore of paramount importance to address promptly.[3]

INTERPRETATION OF OXYGENATION

The A–a gradient can be calculated by subtracting the PaO_2 from the partial pressure of alveolar oxygen (PAO_2). The abbreviation PAO_2 represents the partial pressure of oxygen in the alveoli, which is determined by utilizing the alveolar gas equation. The variable PaO_2 represents the partial pressure of oxygen in arterial blood, specifically determined through the arterial partial pressure of oxygen (PO_2) in the arterial blood A–a gradient.

The A–a gradient can be calculated using the formula: $FiO_2 \times (P_{atm} - PH_2O) - (PaCO_2/0.8)$. The partial pressure of oxygen in arterial blood, commonly referred to as PaO_2, is a critical parameter used to assess the oxygen.

A simplified version of the formula is like this:

$$PAO_2 = (FiO_2 \times 713) - (PaCO_2 \times 1.25)$$

Subtracting PAO_2 from the PaO_2 will give us the A–a gradient.

At sea level, the FiO_2 is 0.21, the atmospheric pressure (P_{atm}) is 760 mm Hg, and the partial pressure of water vapor (PH_2O) is 47 mm Hg. The typical A-a gradient is generally observed to be below 10 mm Hg; however, it may vary within the range of 5–20 mm Hg.

Another expeditious approach to assess oxygenation deficit involves examining the ratio of PaO_2 to FiO_2.

The calculation of the PaO_2/FiO_2 (P/F ratio) involves dividing the arterial PO_2 value obtained from ABG analysis by the FiO_2 value, which represents the fraction (expressed as a decimal) of inspired oxygen that the patient is getting. Typically, the P/F ratio is between 400 and 500 in person breathing room air.

The P/F ratios in acute respiratory distress syndrome (ARDS) are of interest in academic research and clinical practice.

The difference between 300 and 200 might be classified as "mild" ARDS.

The difference between 200 and 100 is classified as "moderate" ARDS.

Patients with a P/F ratio of <100 are classified as having "severe" ARDS.[4,5]

The second step involves evaluating the pH level. The presence of acidosis or alkalosis can be determined by assessing the pH value, which shows the presence of acidemia or alkalemia, respectively. In the event that the pH level is within the normal range, it can be inferred that either there is an absence of any acid–base irregularity or there exists a compensatory disease, with alkalosis, which serves to offset the acidosis.[5]

The third step involves the determination of whether the major impairment is of metabolic or respiratory origin. The clinical evaluation, as well as the correlation between alterations in pH, bicarbonate (HCO_3^-), and partial pressure of arterial carbon dioxide ($PaCO_2$), can provide insights into the etiology of the condition. In cases of primary metabolic illnesses, alterations in pH and $PaCO_2$ exhibit a concordant relationship (change in same direction), but in primary respiratory disorders, changes in pH and $PaCO_2$ demonstrate a discordant relationship (change in opposite directions).[6]

The fourth step involves utilizing either the Boston or the Copenhagen bedside criteria to evaluate the suitability of the compensating response. In the event that the observed

TABLE 1: Normal values of $PaCO_2$, pH, HCO_3^-

	Mean	Range
$PaCO_2$ (mm Hg)	40	35–45
pH	7.4	7.35–7.45
HCO_3^- (mEq/L)	24	22–26

TABLE 2: Expected changes in various conditions.

Respiratory acidosis	pH decreases	Bicarbonate increases	$PaCO_2$ increases
Respiratory alkalosis	pH increases	Bicarbonate decreases	$PaCO_2$ decreases
Metabolic acidosis	pH decreases	Bicarbonate decreases	$PaCO_2$ decreases
Metabolic alkalosis	pH increases	Bicarbonate increases	$PaCO_2$ increases

TABLE 3: Acid–base disorders and their primary and compensatory changes.

Disorders	Primary changes	Compensatory changes
Metabolic acidosis	$[HCO_3^-] < 22$ mmol/L	$PaCO_2$ (mm Hg) = $1.5 \times (HCO_3^-) + 8$ $PaCO_2$ (kPa) = $[(HCO_3^-)/5] + 1$
Metabolic alkalosis	$[HCO_3^-] > 26$ mmol/L	$PaCO_2$ (mm Hg) = $0.7 \times (HCO_3^-) + 21$ $PaCO_2$ (kPa) = $[(HCO_3^-)/10] + 2.6$
Respiratory acidosis (acute)	$PaCO_2 > 45$ mm Hg (6.0 kPa)	HCO_3^- (mm Hg) = $[(PaCO_2 - 40)/10] \times 1 + 24$ HCO_3^- (kPa) = $[(PaCO_2 - 5.3)/4] \times 3 + 24$
Respiratory acidosis (chronic)	$PaCO_2 > 45$ mm Hg (6.0 kPa)	HCO_3^- (mm Hg) = $[(PaCO_2 - 40)/10] \times 4 + 24$ HCO_3^- (kPa) = $(PaCO_2 - 5.3) \times 3 + 24$
Respiratory alkalosis (acute)	$PaCO_2 < 35$ mm Hg (4.7 kPa)	HCO_3^- (mm Hg) = $24 - [(40 - PaCO_2)/10] \times 2$ HCO_3^- (kPa) = $24 - 1.5 \times (5.3 - PaCO_2)$
Respiratory alkalosis (chronic)	$PaCO_2 < 35$ mm Hg (4.7 kPa)	HCO_3^- (mm Hg) = $24 - [(40 - PaCO_2)/10] \times 5$ HCO_3^- (kPa) = $24 - 4 \times (5.3 - PaCO_2)$

compensation deviates from the anticipated normal compensation range, it is probable that multiple acid–base disorders are present **(Table 3)**.[6]

The fifth step should be to mind the gaps.

In the presence of metabolic acidosis, the anion gap (AG) should be calculated.

$$\text{Anion gap} = \{(\text{sodium} + \text{potassium} - (\text{chloride} + \text{bicarbonate}))\}$$

The principle of electrochemical neutrality necessitates that the sum of cations must be equal to the sum of anions. The discrepancy should suggest the existence of unmeasured anions and a typical range for the AG is around 12 ± 4 mmol/L. Albumin, which is classified as a weak acid, is responsible for the majority of unmeasured anions. Consequently, in hypoalbuminemia, the AG is affected, necessitating the need for correction.

$$AG_{corr} = AG + (40 - \text{measured albumin}/4)$$

The presence of an elevated AG is highly indicative of the existence of a primary metabolic acidosis and frequently serves as a valuable indicator for identifying the underlying cause of metabolic acidosis, such as the presence of lactate or keto acids.[7]

The common causes of high anion gap metabolic acidosis (HAGMA) are as follows:
- Diabetic ketoacidosis (DKA)
- Lactic acidosis
- Alcohols
- Renal failure
- Starvation ketoacidosis.

The condition known as normal AG metabolic acidosis is characterized by the presence of acidosis despite a normal AG.[8]

The common causes of normal anion gap metabolic acidosis (NAGMA) are as follows:[9]
- Excessive administration of normal saline
- Carbonic anhydrase inhibitors
- Ureteric fistula

- Renal tubular acidosis (RTA)
- Small bowel fistula.

The presence of two metabolic acid-base problems can be identified by determining the discrepancy between the alteration in AG (ΔAG) and the alteration in serum bicarbonate (ΔHCO_3^-). The aforementioned computation is commonly referred to as either the bicarbonate gap or the delta gap. The bicarbonate (delta) gap can be calculated by subtracting the ΔAG from the change in bicarbonate concentration (ΔHCO_3^-).

The equation for ΔAG is defined as the difference between the patient's AG and the normal AG, which is equal to 12 mEq/L.

The change in concentration of bicarbonate ions (HCO_3^-) in the patient's blood, denoted as delta HCO_3^-, is equal to 26 mEq/L, subtracted from the normal concentration of HCO_3^- in the blood.

Typically, in cases with AG acidosis, the delta gap is observed to be zero. The presence of a positive-elevated delta gap or a lowered delta gap indicates the existence of a mixed lesion.

A delta gap of 6 mEq/L indicates the potential occurrence of metabolic alkalosis and/or retention of HCO_3^-.

A delta gap value below -6 mEq/L indicates the potential presence of hyperchloremic acidosis and/or excessive excretion of HCO_3^-.[10]

The osmolar gap refers to the disparity between the estimated plasma osmolality and the measured osmolality. The disparity is often below 20 mOsm/kg H_2O. If the concentration is elevated, it indicates the existence of unaccounted ions.

The calculation for serum osmolality is derived as follows:

$$2 \times (Na^+) + (glucose)/18 + (BUN)/2.8$$

Where BUN is blood urea nitrogen where all units are measured in mg/dL.

It is important to note that the normal range for serum osmolality is typically between 280 and 290 mOsm/kg H_2O.[11]

The causes of increased osmolar gap are as follows:
- Ethylene glycol
- Mannitol
- Alcohol
- Sorbitol.[10]

CASE SCENARIO 1: ACUTE RESPIRATORY ALKALOSIS

Parameters	Day 1
pH	7.48
PaO$_2$ (mm Hg)	83
PaCO$_2$ (mm Hg)	18
HCO$_3^-$ (mmol/L)	22
Glucose (mg/dL)	98
Lactate (mmol/L)	2.5

***Diagnosis:* Respiratory alkalosis**

Definition
- Respiratory alkalosis is a primary acid–base disorder in which arterial partial pressure of carbon dioxide ($paCO_2$) falls to a level lower than expected.
- If there is a coexisting metabolic acidosis, then the expected $PaCO_2$ used for comparison is not 40 mm Hg but a calculated value, which adjusts for the amount of change in arterial PCO_2, which occurs due to respiratory compensation.

Causes
- Hyperventilation (i.e., increased alveolar ventilation) is the mechanism responsible for the lowered arterial PCO_2 in all cases of respiratory alkalosis.
- This low arterial PCO_2 will be sensed by the central and peripheral chemoreceptors and the hyperventilation will be inhibited unless the patient's ventilation is controlled.

Central Causes (Direct Action via Respiratory Center)
- Head injury
- Stroke
- Anxiety—hyperventilation syndrome (psychogenic)
- Others: Pain, fear, and stress—voluntary
- Various drugs (e.g., analeptics and salicylate intoxication)
- Various endogenous compounds (e.g., progesterone during pregnancy, cytokines during sepsis, and toxins in patients with chronic liver disease).

Pulmonary Causes (Act via Intrapulmonary Receptors)
- Hypoxemia (act via peripheral chemoreceptors)
- Pulmonary embolism
- Pneumonia
- Asthma
- Pulmonary edema (all types).

Maintenance
- Requires a persistent disorder
- This is different from the situation with a metabolic alkalosis where maintenance of the disorder requires an abnormality to maintain it as well as the problem which initiated it.

Effects of Hypocapnia
- Central nervous system
  - Increased neuromuscular irritability (e.g., paresthesias such as circumoral tingling and numbness and carpopedal spasm)
  - Decreased intracranial pressure (secondary to cerebral vasoconstriction)
  - Inhibition of respiratory drive via the central and peripheral chemoreceptors
  - Cerebral blood flow (CBF) decreases quite markedly with hypocapnia
  - Lightheadedness and confusion

- Cardiovascular system (CVS)
  - Cerebral vasoconstriction (causing decreased CBF)
  - Cardiac arrhythmias
  - Decreased myocardial contractility
  - Shift of the hemoglobin oxygen dissociation curve to the left (impairing peripheral oxygen unloading)
  - Slight fall in plasma [K^+].

Compensation

Compensation in an Acute Respiratory Alkalosis

- *Mechanism:* Not really compensation, but changes in the physicochemical equilibrium of the bicarbonate buffer system occur due to the lowered PCO_2, and this results in a slight decrease in HCO_3^-.
- *Magnitude:* Drop in HCO_3^- by 2 mmol/L for every 10 mm Hg decrease in PCO_2 reference value of 40 mm Hg.
- *Limit:* The lower limit of "compensation" for this process is 18 mmol/L, so bicarbonate levels below that in an acute respiratory alkalosis indicate a coexisting metabolic acidosis.

Compensation in a Chronic Respiratory Alkalosis

- *Mechanism:* Renal retention of acid causes a further fall in plasma bicarbonate.
- *Magnitude:* Studies have shown an average 5 mmol/L decrease in [HCO_3^-] per 10 mm Hg decrease in PCO_2 from the reference value of 40 mm Hg.
- *Limit:* The limit of compensation is a [HCO_3^-] of 12-15 mmol/L.

Management

- Hypoxemia is an important cause of respiratory stimulation and consequent respiratory alkalosis—gives O_2.
- The decrease in arterial PCO_2 inhibits the rise in ventilation—the hypocapnic inhibition of ventilation (acting via the central chemoreceptors) may leave the patient with an impaired state of tissue oxygen delivery.
- In most cases, correction of the underlying disorder will resolve respiratory alkalosis.[12,13]

CASE SCENARIO 2: CHRONIC RESPIRATORY ALKALOSIS

A climber is coming down from the summit of Mount Everest. The blood gas at an altitude of 8,400 meters reveals pH 7.55, PCO_2 12, PO_2 30, and HCO_3^- 10.5.

Acid-base Status

- The patient has a high pH (alkalemia).
- The PCO_2 is low (respiratory alkalosis) and the bicarbonate is also low (metabolic acidosis). The high pH in conjunction with the low PCO_2 tells us that the respiratory alkalosis is the primary process.
- Metabolic acidosis is a compensatory process.

Diagnosis: **Primary respiratory alkalosis with metabolic compensation.**[12,13]

CASE SCENARIO 3: ACUTE RESPIRATORY ACIDOSIS

A 24-year-old woman is found on the roadside by some bystanders. The medics are called and, upon arrival, they find her with an oxygen saturation of 88% on room air and pinpoint pupils on examination. She is brought into the emergency room (ER) where a room air ABG is performed that reveals: pH 7.25, PCO_2 60, PO_2 65, HCO_3^- 26, and base excess 1. Her chemistry panel shows: sodium 137, chloride 100, and bicarbonate 26.

Acid–base Status

- The patient has a low pH (acidemia).
- The PCO_2 is high (respiratory acidosis) and the bicarbonate is at the upper end of normal. The low pH and high PCO_2 imply that the respiratory acidosis is the primary process.
- The AG is 10 and is, therefore, normal. The patient does not have elevated AG acidosis.
- There is no compensatory process. Although the measured bicarbonate is just above normal, the base excess of 1 tells us that there is no metabolic alkalosis.
- The delta gap is 10 - 12 = -2 and the delta–delta is -2 + 27 = 25. There is, therefore, no metabolic process.

Diagnosis: **An acute, uncompensated respiratory acidosis leading to acidemia during acute opioid poisoning.**

Respiratory acidosis is caused by CO_2 retention because of various causes, so treatment ensures adequate ventilation. There is no role of sodium bicarbonate in the treatment of respiratory acidosis; in fact, it is contraindicated.[12,13]

CASE SCENARIO 4: CHRONIC RESPIRATORY ACIDOSIS

A 60-year-old man with amyotrophic lateral sclerosis is brought into clinic by his family who are concerned that he is more somnolent than normal. On further history, they report that he has been having problems with morning headaches and does not feel very refreshed when he wakes up. An ABG is performed and reveals: pH 7.37, PCO_2 57, PO_2 70, and HCO_3^- 32.

Acid–base Status

- The patient has a low pH (acidemia).
- The PCO_2 is high (respiratory acidosis) and the bicarbonate is high (metabolic alkalosis). The low pH in combination with the high PCO_2 tells us that the respiratory acidosis is the primary process.
- Metabolic alkalosis is a compensatory process.

Diagnosis: **A chronic respiratory acidosis with a compensatory metabolic alkalosis.**[12,13]

CASE SCENARIO 5: METABOLIC ACIDOSIS

A 75-year-old male patient, with history of fever and drowsiness with reduced oral intake since last 4–5 days, was admitted with severe abdominal pain and persistent vomiting.

8 Acid–base Balance and Disorders and Stepwise Approach to their Interpretation with Case Scenario

ABG sampling reveal pH 7.25, PCO_2 37.5 mm Hg, lactate 1.4 mmol/L, bicarbonate 16.3 mmol/L, glucose 61.2 mg/dL, ketones 3.3 mmol/L, sodium 137 mmol/L, chloride 94 mmol/L, and potassium 4.5 mmol/L.

1. **Can you analyze this blood gas?**

pH	7.15
PCO_2 (mm Hg)	20
Bicarbonate (mmol/L)	8
Blood glucose (mmol/L)	450
Blood lactate (mmol/L)	1.5
Sodium (mmol/L)	136
Potassium (mmol/L)	5.0
Chloride (mmol/L)	102

   Diagnosis: **Metabolic acidosis**
   This is metabolic acidosis with high AG with full respiratory compensation.

2. **What are the causes of high AG acidosis?**
   - *Ketoacidosis:*
     - DKA
     - Alcoholic ketoacidosis
     - Starvation ketoacidosis
   - *Lactic acidosis:*
     - Type A lactic acidosis (impaired perfusion)
     - Type B lactic acidosis (impaired carbohydrate metabolism)
   - *Renal failure:*
     - Uremic acidosis
     - Acidosis with acute renal failure
   - *Toxins:*
     - Ethylene glycol
     - Methanol
     - Salicylates

   This patient is having high AG acidosis with normal blood glucose and elevated serum ketones with history of reduced oral intake, likely cause being starvation ketoacidosis.

3. **What is the pathophysiology of starvation ketoacidosis?**
   Ketoacidosis is a common cause of metabolic acidosis. Ketone bodies (acetoacetate, beta-hydroxybutyrate, and acetone) are produced in liver when hepatic lipid metabolism has changed to a state of increased ketogenesis due to relative or absolute insulin deficiency. During starvation, hepatic glycogen stores are depleted after 12-24 hours of fasting; liver produces ketones to provide energy for peripheral tissues. Ketoacidosis can develop after overnight fasting, but it takes 3-14 days of starvation to reach maximum levels of ketoanion levels.
   Normal ketoanion levels: 1-2 mmol/L

4. **What are the other causes of ketoacidosis?**
   The most common cause of ketoacidosis is DKA. Another cause being alcoholic ketoacidosis along with starvation ketoacidosis.

5. **How to diagnose ketoacidosis?**
   Diagnosis of ketoacidosis is suggested by detection of ketone bodies with high AG metabolic acidosis.
   Differentiation between various causes of ketoacidosis is based on clinical history, severity, and serum glucose levels. Fasting ketosis rarely reduces the bicarbonate level below 17-18 mEq/L.
   Diagnosis of ketoacidosis requires detection of ketone bodies in urine with nitroprusside test or serum with direct assays of beta-hydroxybutyrate levels.

6. **How to manage starvation ketoacidosis?**
   The main cause of ketone production with starvation ketoacidosis is the state of carbohydrate depletion; thus, initial management centers around replacing with intravenous (IV) dextrose. Dextrose will increase insulin secretion and reduce glucagon secretion. This will reduce hepatic fatty acid oxidation and ketones generation. Also, increased insulin levels will inhibit hormone-sensitive lipase in adipose tissues, which leads to reduced fatty acid release.
   Along with carbohydrate replenishment, dyselectrolytemia is equally important. Potassium, phosphate, and magnesium corrections are important as these are electrolytes which will be depleted in patients and as acidosis gets corrected; these will need administration to maintain normal serum values.
   It is important to suspect ketoacidosis in patients with unexplained metabolic acidosis.
   There could be an overlap between starvation ketoacidosis and alcoholic ketoacidosis. Careful monitoring of fluid status and electrolyte is important. When treatment is initiated, patients are at increased risk of hypokalemia because of physiological surge of insulin.[14-17]

CASE SCENARIO 6: LACTIC ACIDOSIS

A 69-year-old patient had a cardiac arrest soon after returning to the ward following an operation. Resuscitation commenced and included intubation and ventilation. Femoral ABGs were collected about 5 minutes after the arrest. ABG done showed pH 7.25, PCO_2 42, PO_2 214, HCO_3 14, lactate 12 mmol/L, and AG 24.

1. **Can you analyze this ABG?**
   Arterial blood gas shows severe metabolic acidosis with high AG with lactic acidosis.

2. **What is the normal value of lactates?**
   - *Normal range:* 0.6-1.8 mmol/L
   - *Hyperlactatemia:* A level from 2 to 5 mmol/L
   - *Severe lactic acidosis:* >5 mmol/L
   - *High mortality with lactate:* >8 mmol/L.

3. **What is the normal physiology of lactate production?**

   Lactate is normally produced by all tissues—major contributors being skin, muscles, red blood cells (RBCs), and brain. All tissues produce lactate under anaerobic metabolism, which enters circulation and is then metabolized by liver and kidney by Cori cycle.

4. **What are the causes of lactic acidosis?**

   Lactic acidosis occurs because of either increased lactate production or impaired lactate metabolism by liver.[5]

   The most common causes of lactic acidosis are enumerated as follows:[6-8]
   - *Type A (tissue hypoperfusion):*
     - Hypovolemia
     - Cardiac failure
     - Sepsis
   - *Type B (decreased utilization):*
     - Alcoholism:
       - ↓ Lactate utilization secondary to hepatic dysfunction
       - ↓ NAD^+/NADH ratio leads to ↑ conversion of pyruvate to lactate
     - Metformin
     - DKA

     Mainly due to D-lactate production, though hypovolemia contributes to:
   - Liver disease (decreased clearance)
   - Adrenergic receptor agonism, namely albuterol, epinephrine, etc.
   - Malignancy
   - Carbon monoxide poisoning
   - Cyanide poisoning
   - *Type D:* Episodes of encephalopathy and metabolic acidosis typically follow high-carbohydrate meals in patients with short bowel syndrome. Type D lactate is not detected with standard lactate levels.

   Sepsis is a very common cause of lactic acidosis in critical care setting.

5. **What are the reasons for increased lactic acid in sepsis?**
   - Endogenous catecholamine release and use of catecholamine inotropes
   - Circulatory failure due to hypoxia and hypotension
   - Microvascular shunting
   - Inhibition of pyruvate dehydrogenase (PDH) by endotoxin
   - Coexistent liver disease
   - Slowed hepatic blood flow—impairing clearance.

6. **What are the reasons for increased lactic acid in sepsis?**
   - Beta-agonists or beta-stimulation
   - Extreme exercise
   - Seizures—immediate postictal period
   - Hepatic failure—lactate ringer's solution unlikely to cause false positive except in hepatic failure.

7. How do you treat lactic acidosis?
- The primary treatment for lactic acidosis is to treat the primary cause and reverse it.
- Maintain good tissue perfusion and maintain adequate oxygenation
- Ensure that patient is hyperventilated to compensate for acidosis
- Use of exogenous bicarbonate is controversial and has not shown any benefit. Best to avoid it, except for treatment of associated severe hyperkalemia
- Hemodialysis may not help in lactate clearance, but it is definitely useful in case of metformin-induced lactic acidosis with high metformin levels (extracorporeal treatment in poisoning).

8. How to manage D-lactic acidosis?
- Along with supportive therapy, the main therapeutic targets are to withdraw contributing factors and reduce enteral carbohydrate intake.
- May consider antibiotic therapy to clear causative bacterial flora
- Refractory cases may require surgery such as small intestine transplant or lengthening procedure.[18-21]

CASE SCENARIO 7: MIXED ACIDOSIS HAGMA + NAGMA

A 20-year-old type I diabetic male came with abdominal pain, persistent vomiting, and high glucose. ABG analysis shows pH 7.05, HCO_3 4.7 mmol/L, Na 139 mmol/L, Cl 114 mmol/L, and AG 20.3 mmol/L and urinary ketones were absent. Signs and symptoms were corresponding to DKA, so the patient was started on DKA regime, but it showed no improvement in the measured parameters nor the patient.

1. **What is the diagnosis?**
   There is metabolic acidosis with high AG. ΔAG is 10.3 and delta bicarb is 19.3. So, the delta ratio is 0.5.
   This suggests that there is AG metabolic acidosis plus non-AG metabolic acidosis.
   Diagnosis: **Mixed AG and non-AG metabolic acidosis**

2. **What is delta gap?**
   Delta gap = (change in AG) – (change in bicarbonate) (It is assumed that the usual AG is 12 and the normal HCO_3 is 24.)
   There is also a condensed equation that does not call for a bicarbonate value:
   $$\text{Delta gap} = Na^+ - Cl^- - 36$$
   The generated ratio's interpretation:
   - –6 = Mixed high and normal AG acidosis
   - –6 to 6 = Only a high AG acidosis exists
   - Over 6 = Mixed high AG acidosis and metabolic alkalosis

   In essence, the delta gap serves as a tool to assess the presence of a typical AG metabolic acidosis. As AG and bicarbonate change simultaneously, delta gap should remain at zero, as that is its normal value. The delta gap will grow increasingly positive, showing the presence of an alkalosis, if the bicarbonate is changing much less than the AG. The delta gap will be very negative if there is acidosis present that is unrelated to the rise in AG and the change in bicarbonate is significantly greater than the change in AG.

3. **What are the limitations of the delta method?**
   Delta gap and delta ratio are based on following assumptions:
   - Acid anions are buffered 1:1 by bicarbonate.
   - All buffering occurs in the extracellular fluid.
   - Acid anions have the same distribution space and clearance mechanisms as the H^+.[22]

4. **What are causes of mixed AG and non-AG metabolic acidosis?**
   Anion gap and non-AG metabolic acidosis can coexist in following setting:
   - *Diarrhea:* In diarrhea, there is usually normal AG acidosis because of bicarbonate loss. But high AG metabolic acidosis can also develop in case of hypoperfusion state, leading to lactic acidosis or reduced renal function, leading to hyperphosphatemia and retention of other organic acids.
   - *Progression of renal diseases:* Kidney disease initially causes normal AG hyperchloremic acidosis, which progresses over a period of time to uremic AG acidosis.
   - *Ketoacidosis:* It causes high AG metabolic acidosis. Along with this normal AG, acidosis can develop in patients with partially treated ketoacidosis or saline resuscitation.
   - In patients with D-lactic acidosis or toluene, toxicity will develop AG acidosis if anion acids are retained or will develop normal AG acidosis if anion acids are excreted.

5. **How to treat mixed AG and non-AG metabolic acidosis?**
   Correction of underlying cause: As much as is possible, the underlying problem should be found and fixed. Unfortunately, addressing the cause of the problem may not be adequate to cause rapid resolution (e.g., in patients with moderate kidney injury).

   Role of bicarbonate: These are conditions which essentially denote bicarbonate deficiency, so giving bicarbonate makes sense physiologically. Exogenous bicarbonate therapy hastens recovery in these patients. Also in uremic acidosis, bicarbonate may be used to treat acidosis and avoid dialysis.

   Bicarbonate can be used as isotonic solution of 1.3% or hypertonic solution of 8.4%.[22-24]

CASE SCENARIO 8: METABOLIC ALKALOSIS

A 68-year-old man has been diagnosed with an acute abdomen. He has been vomiting for the last few days and is dehydrated.

Arterial blood gas analysis shows pH 7.50, HCO_3 36 mEq/L, $PaCO_2$ 44 mm Hg, Na^+ 134 mEq/L, K^+ 2.7 mEq/L, Cl^- 90 mEq/L, and urinary spot chloride <10 mEq/L.

1. **Can you analyze this ABG finding?**
   Metabolic alkalosis: ABG analysis shows metabolic alkalosis with normal AG.
   Predicted PCO_2 is $(0.7 \times HCO_3) + 21 +/- 5 = (0.7 \times 36) + 21 +/- 5 = 46.5$ mm Hg.

Actual PCO$_2$ is 44 mm Hg, so there is no associated respiratory disorder. Urinary chloride is <10 mEq/L, so it is chloride-responsive metabolic alkalosis without respiratory disorder.

2. **What is the etiology of metabolic alkalosis?**
Metabolic alkalosis is usually a temporary process because of high capacity of kidneys to excrete bicarbonate. The persistence of alkalosis requires an initiating process and a maintaining process, which must be considered while analyzing metabolic alkalosis. *The initiating process*:
- Increased alkali within the extracellular fluid (ECF):
  - From an external source (e.g., IV NaHCO$_3$ infusion and citrate in transfused blood)
  - From an internal source (e.g., metabolism of ketoanions to provide bicarbonate)
- Loss of H$^+$ from ECF:
  - Through kidneys (e.g., diuretics)
  - Through gut [e.g., vomiting and nasogastric (NG) suction]

Maintenance of alkalosis: Metabolic alkalosis returns to normal immediately unless there is a process which greatly impairs kidney's ability to excrete bicarbonate. Following are four processes which increase bicarbonate reabsorption from renal tubules or decrease bicarbonate filtration, and thus maintain metabolic alkalosis:
1. Chloride depletion
2. Potassium depletion
3. Reduced glomerular filtration rate (GFR)
4. ECF volume depletion (volume contraction).

3. **What are the causes of metabolic alkalosis?**
Compensatory for a severe, chronic carbon dioxide acidosis

Physiologic response to chronic hypercapnic respiratory failure of any cause, most commonly:
- Severe chronic obstructive pulmonary disease (COPD)
- Obesity hypoventilation
- Chronic respiratory muscle weakness

Chloride-responsive alkalosis (urine chloride <10–30 mm; usually patient is hypovolemic and this responds to saline therapy):
- Vomiting or NG suction
- Chloride-wasting diarrhea (villous adenoma and laxative abuse)
- Remote diuresis
- High-dose Na penicillin therapy
- Renal hypoperfusion (due to hypovolemia, failure, or cirrhosis) plus exogenous alkali:
  - Total parenteral nutrition (TPN) with excess acetate
  - Citrate (massive transfusion and plasmapheresis)
  - Bicarbonate administration (e.g., milk–alkali syndrome and carbonate intake)

Nonchloride-responsive alkalosis (urine chloride >10–30 mm, often unresponsive to saline therapy):
- Active treatment with thiazide or loop diuretics
- Hypomagnesemia or severe hypokalemia

- Hyperaldosteronism of any etiology (may be supported by presence of hypertension):
  - *Primary aldosteronism:* Aldosterone-secreting adenoma and bilateral adrenal hyperplasia
  - *Secondary aldosteronism:* Renin-secreting tumor, high blood pressure, and arteria stenosis
  - Cushing's syndrome and exogenous mineralocorticoid
- Renal insufficiency plus exogenous alkali:
  - TPN with excess acetate
  - Citrate (massive transfusion and plasmapheresis)
  - Bicarbonate administration (e.g., milk-alkali syndrome and carbonate intake).

4. **How to investigate metabolic alkalosis?**
   1. *History and physical (H&P) examination:* Review should tell about the cause of metabolic alkalosis. Hypovolemia denotes chloride-responsive metabolic alkalosis, while hypertension can indicate aldosterone activity.
   2. *Basic laboratory investigations—if cause unclear:*
      - Serum electrolytes (including Ca/Mg/P)
      - Blood gas to assess for compensatory metabolic alkalosis
      - Urine potassium and chloride levels:
        - Urine potassium <20-30 mM suggests that hypokalemia may be contributory.
        - Urine chloride concentration is the most important:
          - Chloride <10-30 mM suggests saline responsive
          - Chloride >10-30 mM suggests saline unresponsive
          - Chloride between 10-30 mM lies in a gray area that does not provide reliable diagnostic information.
   3. *Renin-angiotensin-aldosterone system (RAAS) assessment:* To consider when, urine chloride >10-30 mM or metabolic alkalosis remains unresponsive to normal saline infusion or if there are other clinical features of hyperactive RAAS, such as hypertension and hypokalemia.
      - Low renin and high aldosterone—primary hyperaldosteronism
      - High renin and high aldosterone—secondary hyperaldosteronism
      - Low renin and low aldosterone—state of apparent mineralocorticoid excess.

5. **How to treat metabolic alkalosis?**
   Main principles of therapy are: Correct the primary cause of metabolic alkalosis and also correct the factors which maintain the disorder.
   - If possible, rectify primary disease process (e.g., correct pyloric obstruction and cease diuretics)
   - Fix the reason impairing renal bicarbonate excretion (i.e., give chloride, water, and K^+)
   - Expand ECF volume with normal saline (and KCl if K^+ deficiency)
   - Rarely ancillary measures such as:
     - HCl infusion
     - Acetazolamide (one or two doses only)
     - Oral lysine hydrochloride

- Supportive measures (e.g., give O_2 in view of hypoventilation—appropriate monitoring and observation)
- Avoid hyperventilation as this worsens the alkalemia.[24-27]

REFERENCES

1. Joynt GM, Choi GYS. Blood gas analysis in the critically ill. Oxford Textbook of Critical Care. USA: Oxford Textbook of Critical Care; 2016. pp. 326-30.
2. Hall JE, Guyton AC. Guyton and Hall Textbook of Medical Physiology, 11th edition. Philadelphia, PA: Saunders; 2011.
3. Cooper N. Acute care: Arterial blood gases. Student BMJ. 2004;12:89-132.
4. Haber RJ. A practical approach to acid–base disorders. West J Med. 1991;155:146-51.
5. Williams AJ. ABC of oxygen. Assessing and interpreting arterial blood gases and acid–base balance. BMJ. 1998;317:1213-6.
6. Madias NE, Androgue HJ. Respiratory alkalosis and acidosis. In: Seldin DW, Giebisch G (Eds). The Kidney: Physiology and Pathophysiology, 3rd edition. Philadelphia: Lippincott/Williams & Wilkins; 2000. pp. 2131-66.
7. Fanelli V, Vlachou A, Ghannadian S, Simonetti U, Slutsky AS, Zhang H. Acute respiratory distress syndrome: new definition, current and future therapeutic options. J Thorac Dis. 2013;5(3):326.
8. Adrogué H, Madias N. Management of life-threatening acid–base disorders. N Engl J Med.1998;338(2):107-11.
9. Farkas J. (2019). Non-Anion-Gap Metabolic Acidosis (NAGMA). [online] Available from: https://emcrit.org/ibcc/nagma/ [Last accessed October, 2023].
10. Yee J, Frinak S, Mohiuddin N, Uduman J. Fundamentals of arterial blood gas interpretation. Kidney360. 2022;3(8):1458-66.
11. Emmett M, Nairns RG. Clinical use of anion gap. Medicine (Baltimore). 1977;56(1):38-54.
12. Martinez-Maldonado M, Sanchez-Montserrat R. Respiratory acidosis and alkalosis. Clin Nephrol. 1977;7(5):191-200.
13. Patel S, Sharma S. Respiratory Acidosis. In: StatPearls [Internet]. Treasure Island (FL): StatPearls Publishing; 2023.
14. Emmett M, Szerlip H. (2023). Approach to the adult with metabolic acidosis. [online] Available from: https://www.uptodate.com/contents/approach-to-the-adult-with-metabolic-acidosis [Last accessed October, 2023].
15. Gall AJ, Duncan R, Badshah A. Starvation ketoacidosis on the acute medical take. Clin Med (Lond). 2020;20(3):298-300.
16. Mostert M, Bonavia A. Starvation Ketoacidosis as a cause of unexplained metabolic acidosis in the perioperative Period. Am J Case Rep. 2016;17:755-8.
17. Mehta A, Emmett M. (2023). Fasting ketosis and alcoholic ketoacidosis. [online] Available from: https://www.uptodate.com/contents/fasting-ketosis-and-alcoholic-ketoacidosis [Last accessed October, 2023].
18. Kruse JA, Carlson RW. Lactate metabolism. Crit Care Clin. 1987;3(4):725-46.
19. Nickson C. (2020). Lactate and Lactic Acidosis. [online] Available from: https://litfl.com/lactate-and-lactic-acidosis/ [Last accessed October, 2023].
20. Luft FC. Lactic acidosis update for critical care clinicians. J Am Soc Nephrol. 2001;12 Suppl 17:S15-9.
21. Farkas J. (2021). Metformin toxicity. [online] Available from: https://emcrit.org/ibcc/metformin/ [Last accessed October, 2023].
22. Wrenn K. The delta gap: an approach to mixed acid–base disorders. Ann Emerg Med. 1990;19(11):1310-3.

23. Paulson WD, Gadallah MF. Diagnosis of mixed acid-base disorders in diabetic ketoacidosis. Am J Med Sci. 1993;306(5):295-300.
24. Farkas J. (2021). Metabolic Alkalosis. [online] Available from: https://emcrit.org/ibcc/metabolic-alkalosis/ [Last accessed October, 2023].
25. Emmett M, Szerlip H. Causes of metabolic alkalosis. [online] Available from: https://www.uptodate.com/contents/causes-of-metabolic-alkalosis [Last accessed October, 2023].
26. Mehta A, Emmett M. Treatment of metabolic alkalosis. [online] Available from: https://www.uptodate.com/contents/treatment-of-metabolic-alkalosis [Last accessed October, 2023].
27. Soifer JT, Kim HT. Approach to metabolic alkalosis. Emerg Med Clin North Am. 2014;32(2):453-63.

CHAPTER 2

Common Electrolyte Imbalances

Pramila Chandan, PragnaSree R, Gagana BN, Charudatt Vaity

CASE SCENARIO 1: PSEUDOHYPONATREMIA

A 46-year-old man with familial hypercholesterolemia was admitted with complaints of headache, fever, and malaise.

On admission, his laboratory results obtained were as follows: Sodium 121 mmol/L, potassium 3.9 mmol/L, chloride 81 mmol/L, glucose 122 mg/dL, total protein 4.0 g/dL, albumin 2.6 g/dL, total bilirubin 8.9 mg/dL, blood urea nitrogen (BUN) 31 mg/dL, and alkaline phosphatase 568 U/L. Antimitochondrial antibodies were negative and thyroid-stimulating hormone was normal.

Serum osmolality measured was 292 mOsm/L. On the lipid panel, the triglyceride concentration was 960 mg/dL and cholesterol was 1449 mg/dL.

1. **What is your interpretation?**

   Pseudohyponatremia: It is an uncommonly encountered laboratory abnormality defined by a serum sodium concentration of <135 mEq/L in the setting of a normal serum osmolality (280–300 mOsm/kg). Conversely, true hyponatremia is associated with low serum osmolality and should prompt evaluation for the presence of an additional abnormal solute that may be affecting the laboratory assessment. There are many disease states and conditions attributable to the development of pseudohyponatremia. The most common cause of pseudohyponatremia is due to severely elevated levels of cholesterol. Some sources cite the presence of osmotically active solutes, such as mannitol or hyperglycemia, as an additional etiology of pseudohyponatremia.[1]

   Examples of pseudohyponatremia due to accumulation of cholesterol components include:
   - Hypertriglyceridemia
   - Hyperlipidemia
   - Lipoprotein X accumulation (typically secondary to biliary obstruction or cholestasis, such as primary biliary cirrhosis)
   - Familial hypercholesterolemia.[2]

   Abnormally high levels of protein, including native or exogenous immunoglobulins, may also result in pseudohyponatremia.
   - Chronic infectious disease states, such as the hepatitis C virus or human immunodeficiency virus (HIV)
   - Malignant monoclonal gammopathies, such as multiple myeloma, POEMS (Polyneuropathy, Organomegaly, Endocrinopathy, Monoclonal plasma cell disorder, Skin changes) syndrome, and Waldenstrom macroglobulinemia
   - Malignancy—particularly, malignant lymphoproliferative disorders

- Myelodysplastic syndromes
- Heavy chain disease
- Light chain disease
- Immunoglobulin deposition diseases, such as amyloidosis
- Intravenous immunoglobulin (IVIG) therapy.

Pathophysiology

Approximately, 93% of plasma is composed of water and the remaining 7% is composed of solutes. Most electrolytes, including sodium ions, are almost entirely dissociated in the water component of plasma. To measure the serum sodium level, most laboratory evaluation methods require the technician first to dilute the serum sample, thus necessitating a correction factor of 0.93. These indirect methods of serum sodium measurement have proven to be accurate and valid under standard physiologic conditions. However, in the presence of an abnormally excessive level of additional solute, the ratio of solid to water in plasma is altered unpredictably, leading to inaccurate readings when sodium ions are measured indirectly.

$$\text{Corrected Na}^+ = \text{Measured Na}^+ + [\{[0.21 \times \text{triglycerides (g/L)}] - 0.6\} \times (\text{Na}^+/100)].$$

Laboratory Assessment of Serum Sodium

Management of pseudohyponatremia focuses on the treatment of the underlying disorder.

CASE SCENARIO 2: HYPOOSMOLAR HYPONATREMIA

A 53-year-old male with a history of diabetes, dyslipidemia, and hypertension presented to the emergency department with a 6-day history of weakness, fever, and drowsiness. He was on gliclazide and metformin and was recently started on Mixtard 30 units bd because of poor glycemic control, but he stopped injecting insulin 1 week ago.

On arrival, his temperature was 38.9°C, blood pressure (BP) 96/60 mm Hg, pulse 136 beats/min, low volume respiration 36 breaths/min, deep sighing breathing, and drowsy but arousable. He had the tongue coated, dry mucosa and decreased skin turgor; lungs were clear and heart sounds were normal. The abdominal examination showed mild epigastric tenderness to deep palpation, but there was no rebound tenderness or guarding.

Urinalysis: Glucose 4$^+$, ketones 3$^+$, and nitrite and leukocyte negative

Renal profile: Urea 12 mmol/L and creatinine 136 μmol/L.

Parameters—VBG	Values
pH	7.06
PCO$_2$ (mm Hg)	17
Bicarbonate (mmol/L)	5.6
Blood glucose (mmol/L)	30
Blood lactate (mmol/L)	3.2
Sodium (mmol/L)	130
Potassium (mmol/L)	5.0
Chloride (mmol/L)	102

(VBG: venous blood gas)

1. What is the cause of hyponatremia in this patient?

Hyponatremia hyperosmolar

This is a classic case of diabetic ketoacidosis (DKA), with calculated serum osmolality of 302 mOsm/L.

The most commonly used correction factor is a 1.6 mEq/L (1.6 mmol/L) decrease in serum sodium for every 100 mg/dL (5.6 mmol/L) increase in glucose concentration.[3,4]

Corrected sodium = Measured sodium + [1.6 (glucose − 100)/100].

Thus, corrected sodium is 137.4.

A simplified approach to hyponatremia is given in **Flowchart 1**.

Note: The aim is to stop serious signs and symptoms of hyponatremia; do not correct number or aim to correct sodium to normal values.

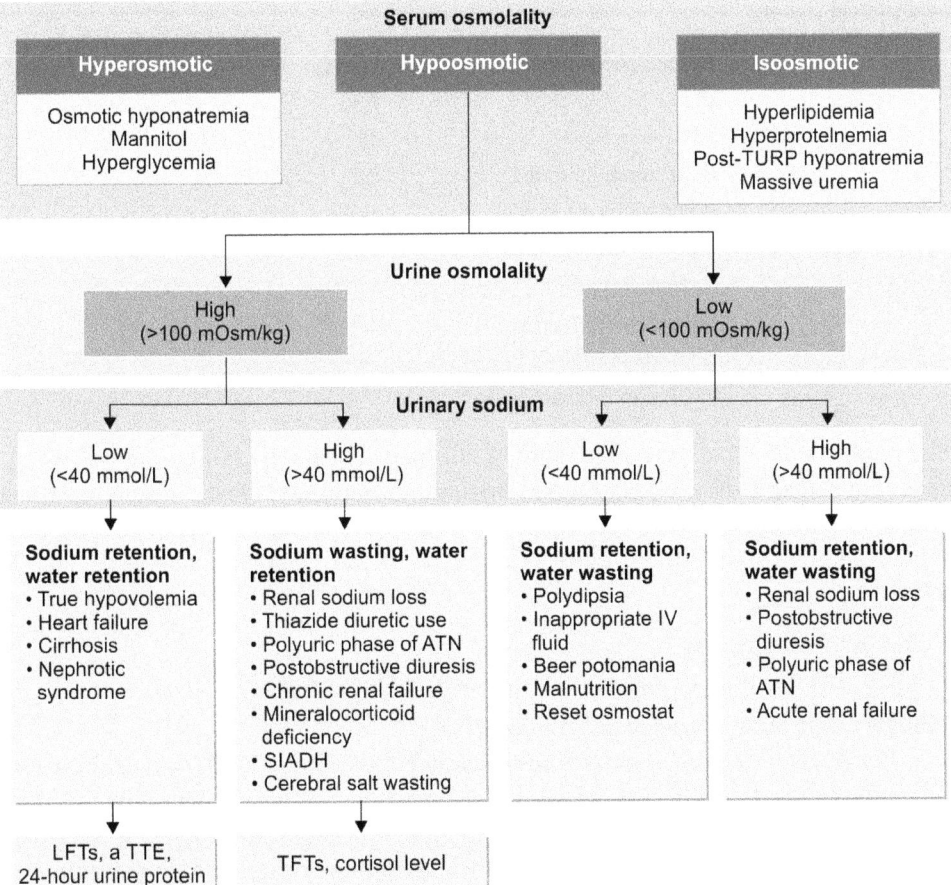

Flowchart 1: Approach to hyponatremia.

(ATN: acute tubular necrosis; IV: intravenous; LFTs: liver function tests; SIADH: syndrome of inappropriate antidiuretic hormone; TTE: transthoracic echocardiography; TFTs: thyroid function test; TURP: transurethral resection of the prostate)

Management Principles

- For active seizures or neurological symptoms, 3% normal saline (NS) can be given initially at 1-2 mL/kg/h, which usually corrects sodium by 1 mmol/L/h. Monitor sodium every 2-4 hourly in such a case.
- Increase in serum sodium by no more than 8-10 mmol/L during first 24 hours of treatment.
- Aggressive correction of 1.5-2 mmol/h for first 3-4 hours with 3% NS is indicated until serious symptoms (such as seizures and obtundation) resolve.
- Sodium deficit = (130 − serum Na) × 0.6 × body weight (in kg)
- 1 liter of 0.9% NS raises serum Na by (154 − serum Na)/[total body water (TBW) + 1].

CASE SCENARIO 3: PSYCHOGENIC POLYDIPSIA

A 34-year-old unmarried woman, a known case of bipolar disorder on medication, presented to casualty with confusion, lethargy, nausea, and ataxia. Venous blood gas (VBG) analysis was done, which showed:

Parameters—VBG	Values
pH	7.36
PCO_2 (mm Hg)	45
Bicarbonate (mmol/L)	24.5
Blood glucose (mg/dL)	120
Blood lactate (mmol/L)	1.2
Sodium (mmol/L)	110
Potassium (mmol/L)	4.0
Chloride (mmol/L)	99

(VBG: venous blood gas)

Her mother stated that the patient started drinking almost 8 L of water per day when her daughter felt sad and/or anxious and had frequent urination. Magnetic resonance imaging (MRI) scan of the brain was normal. Test showed serum osmolality 260 mOsm/kg, urine osmolality 90 mOsm/kg, urine sodium 18 mmol/L, serum creatinine 0.8 mg/dL, and BUN 5 mg%.

1. **What is the diagnosis?**

    Hypoosmolar hyponatremia with dilute urine and low-urine sodium

    This is a case of psychogenic polydipsia (PPD).

    Psychogenic polydipsia or self-induced water intoxication (SIWI) or water intoxication are all used to describe compulsive water drinking. The illness generally develops in three phases, beginning with polydipsia and polyuria, followed by hyponatremia (water is retained as the kidneys fail to excrete the excess fluid, resulting in low sodium serum values), and finally water intoxication, which may manifest as nausea, vomiting, delirium, ataxia, seizures, and coma, and may even be fatal.[5]

Management: Water restriction.

CASE SCENARIO 4: ACUTE TUBULAR NECROSIS

A 45-year-old male, with no known comorbidities, presented with history of fever, nausea, vomiting, and nonbloody diarrhea since 4 days. He presented at 2 PM to casualty and was noticed to not have passed any urine since morning on the day of hospitalization. On examination, he appeared lethargic, drowsy arousable, dehydrated, and showed delayed capillary refill.

His vitals are as follows: Heart rate (HR) 112 beats/min sinus tachycardia, BP 110/70 mm Hg, and respiration rate (RR) 20 breaths/min. The blood investigation showed: Serum creatinine 4.64 mg/dL, BUN 140 mg%, and liver function tests (LFTs) normal. His complete blood count revealed 11,500/mm^3 white cells, 17 g/dL hemoglobin concentration (with hematocrit of 49.8), and 215,000/mm^3 platelets.

Parameters	Day 1
pH	7.32
PaO$_2$ (mm Hg)	132
PaCO$_2$ (mm Hg)	35
HCO$_3^-$ (mmol/L)	16
Glucose (mg/dL)	98
Lactate (mmol/L)	3.5
Sodium (mmol/L)	131
Potassium (mmol/L)	3.2
Chloride (mmol/L)	108
Calcium (mmol/L)	0.89

Renal ultrasound excluded obstructive uropathy with normal-sized kidneys. Urinalysis and microscopy revealed 30 pus cells on high-power field (HPF). He was volume resuscitated and treated for urosepsis. He gradually improved over 48 hours with improving urine output and resolving creatinine; on intensive care unit (ICU) day 3, he again became lethargic, drowsy, arterial blood gas (ABG) showed sudden drop in serum sodium, nurse tells that he has poured 4.5 L of urine in the past 24 hours. The urine osmolarity is low and urine sodium is 45 mmol/L.

1. What is the cause of hyponatremia?

Parameters	Day 1	Day 2	Day 3
pH	7.32	7.38	7.41
PaO$_2$ (mm Hg)	132	128	140
PaCO$_2$ (mm Hg)	35	38	40
HCO$_3^-$ (mmol/L)	16	18	21
Glucose (mg/dL)	98	112	140
Lactate (mmol/L)	3.5	2.1	2.0
Sodium (mmol/L)	140	138	127
Potassium (mmol/L)	3.2	3.8	4.5
Chloride (mmol/L)	108	106	104
Calcium (mmol/L)	0.89	1.15	1.08

Hypoosmolar hyponatremia with dilute urine and high urine sodium

This is hyponatremia in which the normal mechanisms of water resorption and sodium retention have failed.

The usual causes of this state are damaged kidneys, which make no effort to reabsorb sodium [acute renal failure and acute tubular necrosis (ATN)], which fail to respond normally to antidiuretic hormone (ADH). Thus, sodium excretion continues in spite of low sodium, and the urine remains dilute in spite of the fact that there may be hypovolemia.

Polyuric Phase of Acute Tubular Necrosis

Sodium transport in the proximal tubule relies on the action of Na^+/K^+ adenosine triphosphatase (ATPase), maintaining a gradient to drive the Na^+/H^+ antiporter, which gets sodium out of the tubular lumen. In a state of ischemia, this process breaks down and sodium remains in the proximal tubule lumen. Furthermore, they are resistant to aldosterone and ADH. The result is a failure to reabsorb the sodium as it travels down the tubule, as well as a failure to reabsorb water. The resulting urine is likely to be reasonably diluted but with an abnormally high urinary sodium. Replacement with NS seems to be the treatment of choice.[6]

CASE SCENARIO 5: HYPONATREMIA WITH THIAZIDES

A 70-year-old female presented at emergency department with complaints, such as physical weakness, nausea, vomiting, extreme fatigue, and abdominal pain. She was under arterial hypertension treatment with valsartan/hydrochlorothiazide 160/25 mg bd for the past 1 year. On examination, she was drowsy arousable, gave incoherent answers to different questions, BP 150/80 mm Hg, pulse 89 beats/min, SO_2 96%, lungs normal, abdomen soft, liver, spleen, kidneys normal, and no pedal edema.

Head computed tomography (CT) showed no acute lesions. ABG revealed severe hyponatremia with urine osmolarity 212 mOsm/kg and urine sodium 67 mmol/L.

Parameters—ABG	Values
pH	7.49
PaO_2 (mm Hg)	98
$PaCO_2$ (mm Hg)	52
HCO_3^- (mmol/L)	30
Glucose (mg/dL)	108
Lactate (mmol/L)	2.5
Sodium (mmol/L)	104
Potassium (mmol/L)	2.8
Chloride (mmol/L)	77
Calcium (mmol/L)	0.89
(ABG: arterial blood gas)	

1. **What is the diagnosis?**

   Hypoosmolar hyponatremia with concentrated urine–thiazide-induced hyponatremia

   Thiazide diuretics produce volume depletion, which in turn causes ADH secretion, causing water retention, but with ongoing sodium loss, the urine ends up being more sodium rich than the plasma. Unlike the loop diuretics, the thiazides do not impair the medullary osmotic gradient, and ADH can still cause the reabsorption of water into the medulla (whereas the loop diuretics interfere with the medullary gradient, rendering ADH less effective).[7]

CASE SCENARIO 6: SIADH

A 60-year-old male with a known history of small cell carcinoma of lung presents with confusion and lethargy. Clinically, he is euvolemic; serum sodium is 108 mEq/L, K^+ 3.6 mEq/L, serum osmolarity 220 mOsm/kg, urine osmolarity 560 mOsm/kg, urine sodium 47 mmol/L, creatinine 0.8 mg/dL, and BUN 5 mg%; no history of diuretics intake and liver function and thyroid function tests are normal.

1. **What is the diagnosis?**

   Syndrome of inappropriate antidiuretic hormone (SIADH)—tumor-induced

   Diagnostic Criteria for SIADH
   - Hypoosmolar hyponatremia
   - Urine osmolality greater than plasma osmolality
   - Urine sodium excretion >20 mmol/L
   - Normal renal, hepatic, cardiac, pituitary, adrenal, and thyroid function
   - Absence of hypotension, hypovolemia, edema, and ADH-influencing drugs
   - Hyponatremia corrects with water restriction.

   Treatment
   - Water restriction
   - Removal of responsible drugs—diuretics and chlorpropamide
   - Management of physical stress, treat the underlying cause
   - Vasopressin antagonist (Vaptans)—augments free water clearance. SALT II (Study of Ascending Levels of Tolvaptan in Hyponatremia) trial, SALT WATER trial has showed the efficacy and acceptable margin of safety. It is not recommended in acute situations.[8]

CASE SCENARIO 7: HYPERNATREMIA

A 48-year-old female, with 70 kg ideal body weight, underwent total abdominal hysterectomy. On the pouch of Douglas 2 (POD 2), she presented with abdominal distension, vomiting, diagnosed with postoperative ileus, and a Ryle's tube was inserted with continuous suction. 12 hours later, she is obtunded, looks dehydrated, is tachycardic, has BP 100/60 mm Hg, and urine sodium is 9 mmol/L. VBG analysis shows:

Parameters—VBG	Values
pH	7.31
PaO_2 (mm Hg)	40
$PaCO_2$ (mm Hg)	36
HCO_3^- (mmol/L)	18
Glucose (mg/dL)	108
Lactate (mmol/L)	2.5
Sodium (mmol/L)	160
Potassium (mmol/L)	2.8
Chloride (mmol/L)	115
Calcium (mmol/L)	0.89

(VBG: venous blood gas)

1. What is the diagnosis?

Hypernatremia with low extracellular fluid (ECF) indicates that sodium loss is less than water loss, with extrarenal-gastrointestinal (GI) cause in the previous case.

Management

Step 1:

$$\text{Calculation of free water deficit} = \text{TBW} \times [1 - (140 \div \text{serum sodium})]$$

It is based on the assumption that TBW and plasma sodium (PNa) is always constant.

Thus, current TBW × current PNa = normal TBW × normal PNa

Current TBW = (normal TBW × normal PNa) ÷ current PNa

In the above example, for a 70 kg female, normal TBW = 0.5 × 70 kg = 35 L.

Current TBW = (35 × 140) ÷ 160 = 30.5 L

Thus, free water deficit = normal TBW - current TBW = 35 - 30.5 = 4.5 L.

Step 2: Calculation of replacement volume: Free water deficit × 140/sodium in intravenous (IV) fluid.

For example, 1/2 NS contains 77 mEq/L Na.

Thus, replacement volume = 4.5 × 140/77 = 8.1 L.

Sodium correction should always be slow and should not exceed 8–10 mEq/L or 0.5 mEq/L/h

Thus, to correct sodium from 160 to 140, i.e., 20 mEq should occur over 40 h, which means 8.1 L fluid is transfused over 40 h (infusion rate: approximately 200 mL/h).

TBW:
- *Nonelderly male:* 0.6 × patient's weight (in kg)
- *Nonelderly female:* 0.5 × patient's weight (in kg)
- *Elderly male:* 0.5 × patient's weight (in kg)
- *Elderly female:* 0.45 × patient's weight (in kg)

An approach to hypernatremia is given in **Flowchart 2**.[9]

Flowchart 2: Approach to hypernatremia.

Hypernatremia

Hypovolemic — Water loss > Na⁺ loss

- Urinary Na⁺ > 20 mEq/L
  - **Renal loss**
    - Diuretic
    - Glycosuria
    - Renal failure
- Urinary Na⁺ < 10 mEq/L
  - **Extrarenal loss**
    - GI-vomiting
    - GI diarrhea
    - Excessive sweating
    - Respiratory loss

Treatment
- Saline then hypotonic solutions

Euvolemic — Loss of water

- Urinary Na⁺ > 20 mEq/L
  - **Renal loss**
    - Diabetes insipidus
    - Central nephrogenic
- Urinary Na⁺ < 10 mEq/L
  - **Extrarenal loss**
    - Insensible losses
    - Skin respiration

Treatment
- Water replacement
- D5W at 1–2 mEq/L per hour +/− vasopressin for central diabetes insipidus

Hypervolemic — Gain of water and Na⁺

- Urinary Na⁺ > 20 mEq/L
  - **Iatrogenic**
    - Hypertonic NaHCO₃
    - NaCl tablets
    - Hypertonic solutions
  - **Mineralocorticoid**
    - Cushing disease
    - Adrenal
  - **Hypertonic dialysis**
    - Hemodialysis
    - Peritoneal dialysis

Treatment
- Diuretics +/− dialysis

(GI: gastrointestinal)

CASE SCENARIO 8: HYPOKALEMIA

A 41-year-old man with alcoholic liver disease comes to the emergency room (ER) with progressive muscle weakness. VBG analysis shows potassium of 1.9 mEq/L.

Parameters—VBG	Values
pH	7.139
PaO$_2$ (mm Hg)	28
PaCO$_2$ (mm Hg)	37.8
HCO$_3^-$ (mmol/L)	12
Glucose (mg/dL)	108
Lactate (mmol/L)	1.2
Sodium (mmol/L)	139
Potassium (mmol/L)	1.9
Chloride (mmol/L)	115
Calcium (mmol/L)	1.17

(VBG: venous blood gas)

POTASSIUM

It is a major intracellular cation; 98% of total potassium is intracellular and 2% remains in ECF. This concentration gradient is maintained by the sodium–potassium channel. Thus, the change in the serum potassium level does not reflect the actual potassium level change. Potassium is mainly extracted in the urine, whereas a small amount is also excreted in stools and sweat.

Normal potassium in an adult person is 3.5–5.5 mEq/L. The serum potassium level depends on transcellular shift and total potassium loss. Potassium excretion in the kidney depends on sodium reabsorption and aldosterone action.

HYPOKALEMIA

It is defined as the reduction in the serum potassium level of <3.5 mEq/L. The reduction in the potassium level is attributed to transcellular shift, decreased intake, renal loss, and extrarenal losses.

Causes

The causes of hypokalemia are as follows:
- *Transcellular shift:* Intracellular movement of potassium results in low serum level without altering the total body potassium concentration. The factors responsible for the intracellular shift are alkalemia, insulin, beta-agonist, theophylline, refeeding syndrome, hypothermia, thyrotoxicosis, and barium intoxication.
- *Renal loss:* It is seen in cases of diuretic therapy, primary hyperaldosteronism, Cushing syndrome, Liddle's syndrome, and Bartter and Gitelman syndrome. Urinary potassium is >20 mEq/L.
- *Extrarenal loss:* It includes nasogastric suction, vomiting, and diarrhea. Urinary potassium is <20 mEq/L in these cases.

Clinical Manifestations

Mainly asymptomatic few patients may present with generalized muscle weakness and arrhythmias. Electrocardiogram (ECG) changes in hypokalemia are prominent U wave, T flatting, QRS prolongation, prolonged PR interval, and low-voltage complex. Accelerated hypertension is seen in patients with primary hyperaldosteronism and in cases of Cushing syndrome.

Transtubular K gradient (TTKG) is not recommended as per the studies to determine the renal and extrarenal loss of potassium. TTKG < 3 indicates renal conservation. Urinary potassium concentration is used for differentiation of renal from extrarenal loss of potassium.

Management

Potassium replacement: Rapid correction is needed in cases with ECG changes or symptomatic cases. IV replacement under continuous cardiac monitoring should be given (maximun-40 mEq/HR). A dose rate as high as 100 mEq/h can be given safely. Central venous cannula and wide-bored cannulas are preferred for potassium infusion. Potassium chloride is a hyperosmolar solution that needs dilution before administration.

Potassium phosphate solution contains 4.5 mEq/mL potassium and can be used for potassium replacement in severe cases of diabetic ketoacidosis and refeeding syndrome patients. Oral administration is safe and larger doses can be administered safely. Potassium correction should be done with frequent monitoring of the levels. Magnesium supplementation should be considered in refractory cases of hypokalemia.[10]

CASE SCENARIO 9: HYPERKALEMIA

A 70-year-old male, a known diabetic, hypertensive, ischemic heart disease, chronic obstructive pulmonary disease (COPD) patient, comes to ER with breathlessness. He has not been well for the past 1 week and has signs of fluid overload.

Parameters—VBG	Values
pH	7.139
PaO$_2$ (mm Hg)	28
PaCO$_2$ (mm Hg)	37.8
HCO$_3^-$ (mmol/L)	12
Glucose (mg/dL)	108
Lactate (mmol/L)	1.2
Sodium (mmol/L)	139
Potassium (mmol/L)	7.1
Chloride (mmol/L)	115
Calcium (mmol/L)	1.17

(VBG: venous blood gas)

HYPERKALEMIA

Hyperkalemia is defined as a serum potassium level of >5.5 mEq/L. It is a life-threatening condition that requires meticulous correction. The causes are transcellular shift, reduced glomerular filtration, and aldosterone deficiency. Spurious rise in potassium levels is seen in hemolysis sample, leukocytosis, and thrombocytosis.

- *Transcellular shift:* It is the movement of potassium to ECF from intracellular fluid (ICF) with change in total body potassium concentration seen in insulin deficiency, beta-blocker therapy, digitalis intoxication, succinylcholine administration, and hyperkalemia periodic paralysis. Rhabdomyolysis, hemolysis, tumor lysis syndrome, and strenuous exercise cause the release of potassium from cells into ECF. The rise in potassium level with succinylcholine administration is 0.5 mEq/L and its effect is transient, where a rise in potassium levels is high in patients with trauma, burn, and neuromuscular dysfunction.
- *Reduced glomerular excretion:* It is seen in cases with chronic or acute renal disease. Potassium supplementation or intake of potassium-rich foods and blood transfusion in patients with kidney disease causes hyperkalemia.
- *Decreased aldosterone effect:* It seen in patients on angiotensin-converting enzyme (ACE) inhibitors, angiotensin receptor blockers (ARBs), potassium-sparing diuretics,

nonsteroidal anti-inflammatory drugs (NSAIDs), cyclosporine A, type IV renal tubular acidosis, ketoconazole, and pentamidine treatment.

Clinical Manifestation

Clinical manifestation includes neuromuscular weakness that may lead to flaccid paralysis and hypoventilation and cardiac arrest. ECG changes vary widely and may not correlate with the severity of hyperkalemia. This includes tall T wave, mainly in pericardial leads V2 and V3, decreased amplitude of P wave, increased PR interval, widening of QRS complex, and merging of T wave with QRS complex leads to sine wave pattern in severe cases. Ventricular fibrillation and asystole can be seen in severe cases.

Management

The management includes cardiac membrane stabilization activity from the effect of hyperkalemia, augmentation of a transcellular shift of potassium into the cells, and removal of excess of potassium.

- *Membrane stabilization:*
  - *Calcium gluconate:* Calcium antagonizes the depolarization effect of hyperkalemia on cardiac myositis. 10% calcium gluconate is diluted and given slowly and repeated, if necessary, after 5 minutes. It has immediate action, which lasts for 30–60 minutes. Calcium chloride contains three times more elementary calcium than calcium gluconate, but needs central venous access, and can be used in cardiac arrest due to hyperkalemia. Calcium is contraindicated in cases of digitalis toxicity, causing hyperkalemia.
- *Transcellular shift:*
  - *Insulin:* It acts by increasing the uptake of potassium by skeletal muscles via sodium-potassium exchange pump. 10 units of insulin are given with 50% or 25% dextrose. Dextrose is given to counteract the hypoglycemic effect of insulin. Its onset of action is 15 minutes and lasts for 6–8 hours.
  - *Beta-2 agonist:* Albuterol nebulization over 15 minutes at the dose of 10–20 mg is given to potentiate the transcellular shift. Its onset of action is 10 minutes and persists for 3–6 hours. Tachycardia and alteration in blood pressure should be monitored during therapy. IV albuterol 0.5 mg diluted in 100 mL of 5% dextrose can be used.
  - *Bicarbonate:* Bicarbonate infusion at the dose of 2–4 mEq/min can be used till the normalization of potassium level. Effective in patients with normal anion gap metabolic acidosis with hyperkalemia. Short-term infusion has no effect and bicarbonate may form calcium complexes. The side effects include volume overload and hypernatremia.
- *Potassium removal:*
  - *Loop or thiazide diuretics:* They can be used in hyperkalemia and onset of cation lasts for 6 hours. Removal depends on the renal function of the patient.
  - *Cation exchange resin:* Sodium polystyrene sulfonate at the dose of 25–50 mg is given orally of retention enema. It has a slow onset of action and persists for 6 hours. It should be used cautiously in postoperative patients as it increases the chances of intestinal perforation. It is preferred to dilute it with sorbitol.

- *Hemodialysis:* It is the most effective method of potassium removal from the body with immediate onset of action. It is preferred in severe cases with ECG changes and cases which are not responding to medical therapy.[11]

CASE SCENARIO 10: HYPOCALCEMIA

A 35-year-old female with history of parathyroid adenoma postsurgical excision was admitted in the ER with complaints of severe carpopedal spasm, tetany, and abdominal cramps. Initial investigations revealed a serum calcium of 6.4 mmol/L with ionized calcium of 0.99 mmol/L. The rest of the investigations were within normal limits.

1. **What is the diagnosis?**
   Hypocalcemia

   Causes of hypocalcemia
   The list of the causes of hypocalcemia is as follows:
   - *Factitious (most common):*
     - Low albumin
   - *Metabolic (transcellular as for potassium):*
     - Primary respiratory alkalosis (hyperventilation)
     - Chronic alkalosis
   - *Endocrine (decreased Ca uptake and increased excretion):*
     - Reduced parathyroid hormone (PTH) (associated raised PO_4 as cannot excrete)
       - Hypoparathyroidism (raised PO_4)
       - Pseudohypoparathyroidism (raised PO_4)
       - Thyroid or parathyroid surgery
     - Increased calcitonin (decreased Ca and PO_4)
       - Medullary thyroid carcinoma
     - Decreased vitamin D [decreased gastrointestinal tract (GIT) calcium absorption (small)]
   - *Increased phosphate (precipitates calcium in serum):*
     - Tumor lysis syndrome ($\uparrow K^+, \uparrow PO_4, \downarrow Ca^{++}$)
     - Rhabdomyolysis
     - Chronic renal failure
   - *Excessive citrate in circulation (precipitates calcium):*
     - Whole blood transfusion
     - Plasmapheresis
   - *Increased bone formation and turnover (osteoblastic activity):*
     - Malignancy (breast, lung, thyroid, kidney, and prostate)
     - Osteomalacia (increased alkaline phosphatase)
   - *Others:*
     - Sepsis and toxic shock syndrome
     - Pancreatitis (PO_4 normal)
     - Overhydration

- *Drugs:*
  - Beta-blocker od, phenytoin, gentamicin, and heparin
  - Cimetidine and Ca channel blocker.

2. **How do albumin levels affect calcium levels?**
   In patients with chronic illness, malnutrition, cirrhosis, or volume overexpansion, serum albumin may fall with a reduction in the total, but generally not the ionized, fraction of serum calcium. This is referred to as "factitious" hypocalcemia.

   Patients do not have any of the signs or symptoms listed earlier for hypocalcemia. If the serum albumin levels fall to <4.0 g/dL, the usual correction is to add 0.8 mg/dL to the measured total serum calcium for every 1.0 g/dL by which the serum albumin is lowered.

   $$\text{Corrected calcium (mg/dL)} = \text{Measured total calcium (mg/dL)} + 0.8\,(4.0 - \text{serum albumin (g/dL)})$$

   This is not a completely precise method and serum ionized calcium measurements can confirm whether true hypocalcemia is present.

3. **What are the clinical manifestations of hypocalcemia?**
   Calcium is an excitable membrane stabilizer. Neuromuscular excitability and irritability are predominant.
   - *Neurological:*
     - Hyperreflexia and seizures
     - Paresthesia of extremities and face (digital and perioral)
     - Confusion, hallucinations, and dementia
   - *Muscular:*
     - Laryngospasm, stridor, and tetany
     - Muscle spasm, cramps, and tetany
       - Chvostek sign (facial nerve tap—twitch corner of mouth)
       - Trousseau sign (BP cuff on arm for 3 minutes induces carpopedal spasm)
   - *Cardiac:*
     - Decreased myocardial contractility and heart failure
     - ECG changes-QTc prolongation with ST-segment prolongation and T-wave inversion
     - Ventricular tachycardia—Torsades de Pointes
     - Complete heart block

4. **Discuss the management of hypocalcemia**
   - Treat the underlying cause
   - Calcium correction is indicated in:
     - Symptomatic hypocalcemia
     - QT prolongation, in the absence of other causes (e.g., hypokalemia or hypomagnesemia).
     - Severe hypocalcemia (iCa below ~ 0.8 mM)
       Indications for IV calcium therapy are:
       - Symptomatic hypocalcemia
       - Ionized Ca^{2+} < 0.8 mmol/L

- Hyperkalemia
- Ca^{2+} channel blocker overdose
- Hypermagnesemia
- Hypocalcemia with high inotrope requirement
- Massive transfusion
- Postcardiopulmonary bypass

- In severe hypocalcemia, IV calcium is used initially with transition to oral calcium. For mild hypocalcemia, oral calcium could be used for initial treatment.
- IV calcium (10 mL calcium gluconate = 2.3 mmol = 93 mg, 10 mL calcium chloride = 6.8 mmol = 272 mg).

Intravenous loading dose:
- 1 g calcium chloride (if central access) or 2–3 g calcium gluconate (via peripheral line). Either may be infused over 10–20 minutes.
- Calcium chloride can cause tissue necrosis if it extravasates.
- In severe situations (e.g., frank tetany or massive transfusion), this may need to be repeated with careful monitoring of clinical symptoms and iCa levels.
- *Side effects:* Nausea, vomiting, hypertension, flushing, and chest pain.

Intravenous maintenance doses:
- Calcium levels often fall after the initial IV dose, especially if there is a process causing ongoing calcium loss (e.g., pancreatitis).
- Additional smaller doses may be needed (e.g., 1 g calcium gluconate over 60 minutes, repeated hourly).

Oral calcium:
- This may be used for mild hypocalcemia or transitioning patients off IV calcium.
- A reasonable dose of calcium carbonate is 1 g q12h (may escalate to 1 g q6h if needed). Other treatment considerations include correction of hypomagnesemia and hypophosphatemia.[12,13]

CASE SCENARIO 11: HYPERCALCEMIA

A 54-year-old woman with a history of fatigue and midback pain presented to the ER. She had no history of fever, chills, or night sweats but had intentionally lost 27.2 kg in 14 months. She also reported increased thirst during the past month. She had a history of multiple myeloma in her mother. Chest radiography revealed mild curvature of the thoracic spine but was otherwise unremarkable. On examination, her vital signs were as follows: BP 138/74 mm Hg, pulse 85 beats/min, RR 12 breaths/min, and temperature 37.6°C. In general, she appeared in mild distress. Physical examination was unremarkable and her neurologic examination revealed no localizing findings. Results of the initial blood tests were as follows: Hemoglobin 10.4 g/dL, leukocyte count 9.2 × 10^9/L, platelet count 233 × 10^9/L, calcium level 13.9 mg/dL, creatinine level 2.3 mg/dL, BUN level 34 mg/dL, total protein 8.2 g/dL, albumin 3.5 g/dL, and globulin 4.7 g/dL.

1. What is the diagnosis?
Hypercalcemia

Causes of Hypercalcemia
The list of the causes of hypercalcemia is as follows:
- Malignancy (multiple myeloma and metastases to bone)
- Granulomatous disease (tuberculosis and sarcoidosis)
- Endocrine dysfunction (hyperthyroidism, hyperparathyroidism, adrenal insufficiency, and pheochromocytoma)
- Pharmacologic agents (thiazide diuretics, milk-alkali syndrome, PTH therapy for osteoporosis, lithium, and vitamin A)
- Miscellaneous (dehydration, rhabdomyolysis, prolonged immobilization, dietary, and iatrogenic).

2. List the clinical manifestations of hypercalcemia
- Stones (renal colic and hypercalcemic stones)
- Bones (increased osteolysis and fractures)
- Psychic moans (depression, confusion, hallucinations, and coma)
- Abdominal groans (anorexia, nausea and vomiting, constipation, and pancreatitis)
- *Others:*
  - Muscle weakness, malaise, and hyporeflexia
  - Confusion, apathy, and decreased memory
  - Nephrogenic diabetes insipidus (polyuria and polydipsia).

3. What are the ECG changes seen in a patient with hypercalcemia?
- Shortened QT interval
- Osborn waves and notches in the end of the QRS complex (similar to those seen in hypothermia)
- Widened QRS complexes
- Atrioventricular (AV) block.

4. Discuss the management of hypercalcemia
- *Supportive care:* Airway, breathing, and circulations (ABCs), IV, O_2, monitor
- *Volume expansion:* NS administration:
  - *Mechanism of action:* Corrects volume-depleted state and inhibits proximal tubule calcium resorption
  - Monitor other electrolytes (potassium and sodium)
  - *Dose:* Bolus to correct hypotension and careful administration while monitoring overall fluid status (patients often have cardiac and/or renal dysfunction making them susceptible to volume overload)
- *Loop diuretics (i.e., furosemide):*
  - *Mechanism of action:* Inhibits reabsorption of Na, K, and Cl via the $Na^+ - K^+ - 2Cl^-$ cotransporter in the ascending loop of Henle, thereby also inhibiting Ca^{2+} and Mg^{2+} reabsorption.
  - Theoretical benefit of "forced diuresis" is not proven in the literature.

- Should not be given until volume repletion is completed as it can exacerbate hypercalcemia.
- *Bisphosphonates:*
  - *Mechanism of action:* Inhibit osteoclast-mediated bone resorption
  - *Zoledronic acid:* Preferred in hypercalcemia in the setting of malignancy
  - *Dose:* 4 mg IV over 15 minutes
  - *Other agents:* Pamidronate and etidronate
- *Calcitonin:*
  - *Mechanism of action:* Inhibits Ca^{2+} absorption in the intestines, inhibits osteoclast activity, stimulates osteoblastic activity, and inhibits renal tubular cell reabsorption
  - *Dose:* 4 IU/kg intramuscular (IM) q12h
- *Cinacalcet:*
  - *Mechanism of action:* Increases the sensitivity of Ca^{2+} receptors on parathyroid cells to reduce PTH levels and, thus Ca^{2+} levels.
  - *Indications:* Hypercalcemia in patients with secondary hyperparathyroidism [i.e., chronic kidney disease (CKD) on dialysis and parathyroid carcinoma]
- *Other:*
  - Hemodialysis
  - Parathyroidectomy may be considered in patients with hypercalcemia caused by hyperparathyroidism.[14,15]

CASE SCENARIO 12: HYPOPHOSPHATEMIA

A 19-year-old female with history of anorexia nervosa is admitted to hospital with extreme malaise and weakness. Her body mass index (BMI) was 16 kg/m² and was started on enteral feeding via nasogastric (NG) tube. 24 hours later, the patient developed acute-onset breathlessness with type 1 respiratory failure and was shifted to the ICU, requiring intubation after a failed noninvasive ventilation (NIV) trial. Her laboratory findings are as follows:

Na^+	135 mEq/L
K^+	2.3 mEq/L
Cl^-	110 mEq/L
HCO_3^-	25 mEq/L
PO_4^-	1.2 mmol/L
Mg^{+2}	0.7 mmol/L

1. **What do you infer from the above results and what is your initial impression?**

   The patient has severe electrolyte disturbance including hypophosphatemia, hypomagnesaemia, and hypokalemia. In the background of anorexia nervosa and initiation of enteral feeds and associated dyselectrolytemia, diagnosis of refeeding syndrome is most likely.

   Causes of Hypophosphatemia
   The list of the causes of hypophosphatemia is as follows:

- *Inadequate intake or absorption:* Malnutrition, phosphate-binding antacids, vitamin D deficiency, chronic diarrhea, and malabsorption syndromes
- *Redistribution into cells:* Refeeding syndrome and insulin administration in DKA
- *Renal losses:* Diuretic therapy, osmotic diuresis, hyperparathyroidism, and proximal renal tubular dysfunction (Fanconi syndrome)
- *Extreme catabolic states:* Burns, trauma, and sepsis

2. **What is refeeding syndrome and its pathophysiology?**

   Refeeding syndrome describes a constellation of metabolic disturbances that occur as a result of reinstitution of nutrition to patients who are starved or severely malnourished.

   It occurs secondary to switch from lipid and fatty acid metabolism of starvation back to carbohydrate metabolism upon feeding. This results in release of insulin causing intracellular shift of potassium, magnesium, and phosphate, leading to life-threatening multiorgan dysfunction.

3. **What are the risk factors for refeeding syndrome?**

   Risk factors include:
   - Low BMI <18.5 kg/m^2
   - Unintentional weight loss of >5-10% body weight
   - Starvation for >5 days
   - Chronic alcoholism
   - Malignancy postchemotherapy
   - Malabsorption disorders

4. **List of the clinical manifestations noted in refeeding syndrome.**
   - *Cardiovascular system (CVS):* Heart failure, hypotension, shock, and cardiac arrythmias
   - *GIT:* Deranged liver function test (LFT), diarrhea, and delayed gastric emptying
   - *Renal:* Acute tubular necrosis
   - *Respiratory support (RS):* Respiratory muscle weakness and ventilator dependence
   - *Hematological:* Hemolysis and poor platelet function
   - *Musculoskeletal (MSK):* Rhabdomyolysis and tetany
   - *Central nervous system (CNS):* Seizures, delirium, coma, and Wernicke's encephalopathy
   - *Immunological:* Phagocyte dysfunction and increased susceptibility to sepsis

5. **How do you manage refeeding syndrome?**

   Three components fundamental to management of refeeding syndrome (RFS) are:
   - Early identification of at-risk individuals
   - *Monitoring during refeeding:*
     - *Clinical monitoring:* BP, HR, feeding rate, weight gain, fluid balance, and neurological monitoring
     - *Biochemical monitoring:* Electrolyte levels (PO$_4^-$, Mg^{+2}, K$^+$, and Na$^+$), blood glucose levels, and account other sources of energy (dextrose and propofol)
   - *Appropriate feeding regime:*
     - Start with a low-calorie rate of 5-10 kcal/kg/day and gradually build up to 25/kcal/kg/day over a period of 7-10 days with vigorous electrolyte correction as needed

and supplementation of thiamine, vitamin B complex, and trace minerals while maintaining equal fluid balance.
- In case of suspected RFS or intolerance to feed, the energy intake should be stopped or reduced.[16,17]

CASE SCENARIO 13: HYPERPHOSPHATEMIA

A 45-year-old male presented to the ER with complaints of severe muscle cramps and decreased urine output since the last 3 days. He is otherwise a known case of hypertension and nonoliguric CKD on medical management. His preliminary blood investigations revealed the following: hemoglobin 7.8 g/dL, leukocyte count 6.4×10^9/L, platelet count 324×10^9/L, calcium level 13.9 mg/dL, creatinine level 8.3 mg/dL, BUN level 87 mg/dL, sodium 136 mEq/L, potassium 5.95 mEq/L, chloride 102 mEq/L, total protein 6.2 g/dL, albumin 2.0 g/dL, and globulin 4.2 g/dL. Serum phosphorus concentration was markedly increased at 8.4 mg/dL (3.0–4.5 mg/dL).

1. **What is the diagnosis?**
   Hyperphosphatemia

   Causes of Hyperphosphatemia
   The causes of hyperphosphatemia are as follows:
   - Renal failure—most common cause
   - Increased renal resorption (hypoparathyroidism and thyrotoxicosis)
   - Cellular injury with release (tumor lysis syndrome, rhabdomyolysis, hemolysis, and ischemic gut)
   - Medication related—phosphate-containing laxatives, excessive administration, and bisphosphonate therapy.

2. **What are the clinical features of hyperphosphatemia?**
   Most clinical manifestations are due to associated hypocalcemia produced by:
   - Precipitation with calcium (leading to nephrolithiasis)
   - Interference with parathyroid hormone-mediated resorption of bone
   - Decreased vitamin D levels—manifestations of hypocalcemia include muscle cramping, tetany, hyperreflexia, and seizures as well as cardiovascular manifestations, such as prolonged QT.

3. **How do you manage hyperphosphatemia?**
   Hyperphosphatemia can be managed by:
   - Limiting phosphate intake
   - Enhancing urinary phosphate excretion:
     • In the absence of end-stage renal disease, phosphate excretion can be optimized with saline infusion and diuretics—diuretics that work on the proximal tubule, such as acetazolamide, are particularly effective for enhancing phosphate excretion.
     • Any patient with life-threatening hyperphosphatemia should receive dialysis.

- *Oral phosphate binders:* Calcium and aluminum salts are widely used; however, calcium salts may produce metastatic calcification and aluminum salts are toxic.
- In dialysis patients, chronic management with calcium-free phosphate binders such as sevelamer hydrochloride may reduce long-term mortality.[18,19]

REFERENCES

1. Theis SR, Khandhar PB. Pseudohyponatremia. In: StatPearls [Internet]. Treasure Island (FL): StatPearls Publishing; 2022.
2. Song L, Hanna RM, Nguyen MK, Kurtz I, Wilson J. A novel case of pseudohyponatremia caused by hypercholesterolemia. Kidney Int Rep. 2018;4(3):491-3.
3. Huffman GB. Adjusting sodium levels in patients with hyperglycemia. Am Fam Physician. 1999;60(6):1821.
4. Castle-Kirszbaum M, Kyi M, Wright C, Goldschlager T, Danks RA, Parkin WG. Hyponatraemia and hypernatraemia: disorders of water balance in neurosurgery. Neurosurg Rev. 2021;44(5):2433-58.
5. Bhatia MS, Goyal A, Saha R, Doval N. Psychogenic polydipsia—management challenges. Shanghai Arch Psychiatry. 2017;29(3):180-3.
6. Hanif MO, Bali A, Ramphul K. Acute Renal Tubular Necrosis. [Updated 2023 Jul 4]. In: StatPearls [Internet]. Treasure Island (FL): StatPearls Publishing; 2023 Jan. Available from: https://www.ncbi.nlm.nih.gov/books/NBK507815/
7. Hwang KS, Kim GH. Thiazide-induced hyponatremia. Electrolyte Blood Press. 2010 Jun;8(1):51-7. Erratum in: Electrolyte Blood Press. 2012 Dec;10(1):35-6.
8. Padhi R, Panda BN, Jagati S, Patra SC. Hyponatremia in critically ill patients. Indian J Crit Care Med. 2014;18(2):83-7.
9. Manual of Medicine. (2021). Hyponatremia and Hypernatremia in the Emergency Department. Available from: https://manualofmedicine.com/topics/acid-base-electrolytes/hyponatremia-and-hypernatremia-emergency-department/ [Last accessed July, 2023].
10. Kardalas E, Paschou SA, Anagnostis P, Muscogiuri G, Siasos G, Vryonidou A. Hypokalemia: a clinical update. Endocr Connect. 2018;7(4):R135-R146.
11. Dépret F, Peacock WF, Liu KD, Rafique Z, Rossignol P, Legrand M. Management of hyperkalemia in the acutely ill patient. Ann. Intensive Care. 2019;9(1):32.
12. Schafer AL, Shoback DM. Hypocalcemia: Diagnosis and Treatment. In: Feingold KR, Anawalt B, Boyce A, et al. (Eds). South Dartmouth (MA): MDText.com, Inc.; 2000.
13. Nickson C. (2020). Hypocalcaemia. [online] Available from: https://litfl.com/hypocalcaemia/ [Last accessed July, 2023].
14. Maier JD, Levine SN. Hypercalcemia in the intensive care unit: a review of pathophysiology, diagnosis, and modern therapy. J Intensive Care Med. 2015;30(5):235-52.
15. Farkas J. (2023). Hypercalcemia. [online] Available from: https://emcrit.org/ibcc/hypercalcemia/ [Last accessed July, 2023].
16. Khan LU, Ahmed J, Khan S, Macfie J. Refeeding syndrome: a literature review. Gastroenterol Res Pract. 2011;2011:410971.
17. Mehanna HM, Moledina J, Travis J. Refeeding syndrome: What it is, and how to prevent and treat it. BMJ. 2008;336(7659):1495-8.
18. Goyal R, Jialal I. Hyperphosphatemia. In: StatPearls. Treasure Island (FL): StatPearls Publishing; 2022.
19. Nickson C. (2020). Hyperphosphataemia. [online] Available from: https://litfl.com/hyperphosphataemia/[Last accessed July, 2023].

CHAPTER

Case Scenarios and Interpretations of their Investigations

Hamza Dalal, Nachiket Desai, Hozefa Runderawala, Haresh Dodeja, Bindu Mulakavalupil

3.1: ANEMIAS

CASE SCENARIO 1: MICROCYTIC ANEMIA

You are asked to review an 82-year-old gentleman admitted for chest pain and breathlessness on exertion, which has gradually worsened since past 2 months. He has developed mild swelling on both the legs since last 10 days. He has a history of 5 kg weight loss in 3 months. He has no history of jaundice and has never required blood transfusion in the past. He has no history of bleeding from any site. He is a known case of hypertension and ischemic heart disease (underwent angioplasty 2 years hence). He is on regular antihypertensives and antiplatelet agents for his condition.

He was evaluated in the emergency room (ER) and shifted to the intensive care unit (ICU) in view of ST-T changes and suspected acute coronary syndrome.

His vital signs were as follows: Heart rate 110 beats/min, blood pressure (BP) 150/90 mm Hg, respiration rate (RR) 28 breaths/min, and oxygen saturation (SpO_2) 100% on room air. His temperature was 36.8°C. He had severe pallor and mild bilateral pedal edema. The rest of the examination was unremarkable.

His complete blood count (CBC) report was as follows:

		Units	Reference values
Hemoglobin	4.8	g/dL	13–17
Packed cell volume (hematocrit)	18	%	40–50
Red blood cell (RBC) count	3.2	Million/µL	4.5–5.5
Mean corpuscular volume (MCV)	62	fL	83–101
Mean corpuscular hemoglobin (MCH)	24	pg	27–32
Mean corpuscular hemoglobin concentration (MCHC)	28	g/dL	31.5–34.5
Red cell distribution width (RDW)	22	%	11.6–14
Total leukocyte count	6.5	Thousand/µL	4–10
Neutrophil	80	%	40–80
Lymphocyte	18	%	20–40
Monocyte	2	%	2–10
Basophil	0	%	0–1
Eosinophil	0	%	1–6
Platelet count	4.8	Lakh/µL	150–410
Mean platelet volume	9	fL	6.8–10.9

1. **How do you define a patient with anemia and what are the standard methods for measurement of hemoglobin?**

   Anemia is defined in an adult male as hemoglobin value <13.0 g/dL and in an adult female as 12.0 g/dL.

   Hemoglobin value <7 g/dL is considered to be severe anemia as these patients have worsened cardiac outcomes without packed red blood cells (PRBC) transfusion.

   In terms of hematocrit (HCT), values <40 in males and 35 in females qualify as anemia.

   Normal red blood cell (RBC) count in an adult male is 4.5–5.5 million/dL in males and 3.5–4.5 million/dL in females.

   Standard methods to measure hemoglobin are as follows:
   - *Change in color based:*
     - Sahli's method—old and outdated
     - Cyanmethemoglobin method—uses Drabkin's reagent (universally standardized)
     - World Health Organization (WHO) color scale method—for field hemoglobin testing
   - *Change in specific gravity based:*
     - Copper sulfate method
   - *Point of care systems:*
     - HemoCue method/DiaSpect method: Vanzetti's azide hemoglobin method
   - *Automated hematology analyzer:* Cells are counted depending on the size of cells as blood cells are passed through an orifice using an electric current.[1]

2. **What are the RBC indices and what is their utility in classifying a patient with anemia?**

   The red cell indices are mean corpuscular volume (MCV), mean corpuscular hemoglobin (MCH), mean corpuscular hemoglobin concentration (MCHC), and red cell distribution width (RDW).[2,3]

   These indices are calculated by automated hematology analyzers and are widely used to subclassify anemia.
   - *Mean corpuscular volume:* It is the keystone to classify and further evaluate patients with anemia.
     - MCV: HCT/RBC count
   - *Mean corpuscular hemoglobin and mean corpuscular hemoglobin concentration:* These are used to classify patients into hypochromic or normochromic anemia.
     - MCH: Hemoglobin/RBC count
     - MCHC: Hemoglobin/MCV × RBC count
       The only clinical applicability of the MCHC is to identify hereditary spherocytosis, which is the only condition with microcytosis with hyperchromia (MCHC >36 g/dL).
   - *Red cell distribution width:* It helps to identify the degree of anisocytosis in the peripheral blood.
     - The RDW is derived from pulse-height analysis and can be expressed either as the standard deviation (SD) in femtoliter or as the coefficient of variation (CV) (as a percentage) of the measurements of the red cell volume.

- The major utility of the RDW is to distinguish anemia due to iron deficiency and thalassemia minor.
- In the above mentioned patient, MCV is 62 indicating the presence of microcytosis. MCH and MCHC are both low suggestive of hypochromia.

3. **What are the causes of microcytic hypochromic anemia and how would you further evaluate this patient?**

   The differential diagnosis of a patient with microcytic hypochromic anemia is:
   - Iron deficiency anemia
   - Hemoglobinopathy—alpha and beta thalassemia
   - Anemia due to chronic illness
   - Sideroblastic anemia
   - Lead poisoning

   This patient needs an iron study with serum ferritin estimate and a high-performance liquid chromatography to rule out beta-thalassemia.

   In case of a compatible clinical background, alpha thalassemia and sideroblastic anemia can be identified by genetic testing and bone marrow biopsy.

   The presence of multiorgan involvement with characteristic blue lines on gums warrant evaluation for lead poisoning with serum and urinary lead level.

   Anemia due to chronic illness/inflammation is a diagnosis of exclusion.

4. **How do you assess iron status of the body?**

   The iron status of the body can be assessed by the following methods:
   - *Blood tests:* Serum ferritin, serum iron study, total iron-binding capacity (TIBC), transferrin saturation, and soluble transferrin receptor (sTFR) levels
   - *Tissue iron stores:* Bone marrow aspiration/biopsy with Perl's stain

   Ferritin is the storage form of iron. Ferritin levels <50 mg/L indicate depletion of iron stores and a level <15 mg/L is suggestive of clinical iron deficiency anemia.

   In patients with inflammatory disorders, serum ferritin can be high despite tissue level iron deficiency.

   Serum iron levels, TIBC, and transferrin saturation provide a true picture of iron deficiency in patients with inflammatory disorders.

   Transferrin saturation is an accurate test for clinical iron deficiency and levels <10% warrant correction with iron supplementation.

   Soluble transferrin receptor levels are the gold standard to differentiate iron deficiency from anemia due to chronic inflammation. Unfortunately, it is available only as a research tool at present.

   Tissue level iron deficiency can be identified via biopsy of the bone marrow or the liver. Perl's staining of the bone marrow allows grading of iron stores and it has excellent correlation with serum ferritin levels in patients without inflammatory disorders.

5. **Will you advise any further special tests for this patient?**

   As per the rule of the thumb, any elderly male and postmenopausal female with documented iron deficiency should undergo an upper plus lower gastrointestinal (GI) endoscopy to rule out an occult GI blood loss due to a malignancy.

In younger male patients, evaluation to rule a gastric or peptic ulcer is warranted in case other obvious clinical signs of nutritional deficiency are absent.

In female patients in the reproductive age group, menstrual history is of great significance and ultrasound evaluation of uterus and ovaries quite often reveals the underlying cause of excessive menstrual blood loss.

CASE SCENARIO 2: MACROCYTIC ANEMIA

You are asked to review a 24-year-old female patient admitted with complaints of excessive fatigability, hair fall, and jaundice since 1 month. She has no other comorbidities but gives a history of reduced appetite due to oral ulcers. She follows a strictly vegetarian diet. No history of fever or passage of reddish urine.

She was evaluated elsewhere and referred to a higher center in view of severe anemia and thrombocytopenia.

His vital signs were as follows: Heart rate 120 beats/min, BP 100/70 mm Hg, RR 28 breaths/min, and SpO_2 100% on room air. His temperature was 36.8°C. She was cachexic and had severe pallor and mild icterus. She had friable hair and multiple oral ulcers.

His CBC report was as follows:

		Units	Reference values
Hemoglobin	3.6	g/dL	13–17
Packed cell volume (hematocrit)	14	%	40–50
Red blood cell (RBC) count	1.8	Million/μL	4.5–5.5
Mean corpuscular volume (MCV)	128	fL	83–101
Mean corpuscular hemoglobin (MCH)	22	pg	27–32
Mean corpuscular hemoglobin concentration (MCHC)	25	g/dL	31.5–34.5
Red cell distribution width (RDW)	20	%	11.6–14
Total leukocyte count	3.2	Thousand/μL	4–10
Neutrophil	50	%	40–80
Lymphocyte	45	%	20–40
Monocyte	4	%	2–10
Basophil	0	%	0–1
Eosinophil	1	%	1–6
Platelet count	0.65	Lakh/μL	150–410
Mean platelet volume	9	fL	6.8–10.9

1. **How do you interpret the above mentioned report?**
   Macrocytic anemia

   The patient has presented with pancytopenia with severe anemia. The RBC indices are suggestive of macrocytic hypochromic anemia. There is increase in RDW, indicative of anisocytosis.

Severe anemia is also associated with mild leukopenia and thrombocytopenia. The differential count shows normal distribution without obvious atypical cells.

2. **What are the differentials for a patient with macrocytic anemia and how would you further evaluate this patient?**
   Macrocytosis is indicated by an MCV >100 fL in an anemic patient.

   The important differential diagnoses to be considered in this patient are as follows:
   - Megaloblastic anemia—due to vitamin B_{12} or folic acid deficiency[4,5]
   - Aplastic anemia
   - Acute leukemia
   - Myelodysplastic syndrome
   - Hypersplenism.

3. **How do you evaluate a patient with suspected megaloblastic anemia?**
   Megaloblastic anemia is a condition characterized by nuclear-cytoplasmic dissociation affecting the bone marrow precursor cells. The most common cause of this is due to vitamin B_{12} and folic acid deficiencies.

   Evaluation for megaloblastic anemia encompasses the following:[6]
   - A careful peripheral smear examination
   - *Biochemical tests to demonstrate intramedullary hemolysis due to N:C desynchrony:*
     - *High lactate dehydrogenase (LDH):* This level may be disproportionately high (usually >1,000)
     - *Indirect hyperbilirubinemia:* It is generally mild (rarely >3 mg/dL)
     - Low/normal haptoglobin level
     - Reticulocytopenia
   - *Biochemical tests to document vitamin B_{12} or folic acid deficiency:*
     - *Vitamin B_{12} levels:*
       - <200: Considered to be severe deficiency
       - 200–300: Borderline levels
       - >300: Normal
     - *Few caveats about vitamin B12 level testing:*
       - Falsely high if patient has received parenteral B_{12} supplementation.
       - Falsely high in conditions such as myeloproliferative neoplasm due to increase in haptocorrin levels secondary to expanded myeloid cell population.
       - Vitamin B_{12} levels may also be elevated in conditions causing hepatocellular injury such as cirrhosis, hepatocellular carcinoma (HCC), and viral hepatitis due to excessive release of hepatic B_{12} stores into the blood.
       - There is no role for active B_{12} levels in routine diagnosis of vitamin B_{12} deficiency.
     - *Folic acid level:* Serum folic acid level <5 is considered to be associated with clinical folic acid deficiency.
       Red cell folate levels are more accurate measures of cellular folic acid deficiency but not routinely available.

- *Serum methylmalonic acid and serum homocysteine level:*
  - Highly sensitive functional tests to determine cellular deficiencies of vitamin B_{12} and folic acid.
  - These are very useful to enable nutrient supplementation in cases where serum vitamin levels are misleading.
- *Serum haptocorrin levels:* These are useful in cases of myeloproliferative neoplasm.
  - *Bone marrow aspiration/biopsy:* Routine cases of suspected megaloblastic anemia should not undergo a bone marrow biopsy.
    Bone marrow biopsy is reserved for patients who are elderly to rule out myelodysplastic syndrome and for those in whom cytopenias do not recover after adequate vitamin supplementation.

Serum LDH level is an easy tool to identify patients with megaloblastosis even if vitamin levels are inconclusive. Very high LDH levels are seen almost exclusively in megaloblastic anemia.

4. **How to identify the cause of megaloblastic anemia?**
   In our country, dietary factors are the most common cause of vitamin B_{12} deficiency. An exclusively vegetarian diet depletes body B_{12} stores within 2–3 years, leading to clinical deficiency.

   Folic acid stores are depleted much more rapidly (within 2–3 months), especially during periods of increased requirement such as adolescence, pregnancy, and patient with chronic hemolytic anemia.

   Patients who follow a mixed diet and those patients with recurrent megaloblastic anemia should be evaluated further to rule out malabsorption syndromes.

   We routinely advise anti-intrinsic factor immunoglobulin G (IgG) antibody and upper GI endoscopy to rule out pernicious anemia.

   Workup for celiac disease and ileocecal tuberculosis is recommended in patients presenting with a compatible clinical picture.

   One should not forget to do a comprehensive stool examination to rule out worm infestation, especially in younger patients with clinical nutrient deficiency.

5. **What are the causes of macrocytosis in the absence of megaloblastic anemia?**
   Nonmegaloblastic macrocytic anemia can result from a variety of clinical conditions namely:
   - Chronic alcohol abuse
   - Chronic liver disease
   - Bone marrow failure syndromes
   - Myelodysplastic syndromes

   Alcohol by itself can induce RBC macrocytosis even in the absence of liver disease. An ultrasound evaluation of the liver is warranted in all cases to rule out chronic liver disease.

   High index of suspicion of myelodysplastic syndrome should be kept, especially in patients who are older than 60 years as morphological features of myelodysplastic syndrome may closely mimic megaloblastic anemia. Bone marrow evaluation including a conventional karyotyping and next-generation sequencing testing is recommended for identification of this disorder.

CASE SCENARIO 3: NORMOCYTIC ANEMIA

You are asked to review a 64-year-old gentleman admitted for back pain since 1 month. He also complains of increased fatigue and weight loss since 3 months. He presented to ER with sudden intractable back pain, followed by inability to move both lower limbs. Magnetic resonance imaging (MRI) revealed compression fracture of D12 vertebra with destruction of vertebral body with associated soft tissue density—suspected tuberculous involvement.

He is a known case of diabetes and hypertension. He was diagnosed with diabetic nephropathy 1 year back.

His vital signs were as follows: Heart rate 90 beats/min, BP 140/90 mm Hg, RR 28 breaths/min, and SpO_2 100% on room air. His temperature was 38.1°C. He had pallor and spinal tenderness. Neurological examination revealed paraparesis.

His CBC report was as follows:

		Units	Reference values
Hemoglobin	8.5	g/dL	13–17
Packed cell volume (hematocrit)	29	%	40–50
Red blood cell (RBC) count	3.8	Million/µL	4.5–5.5
Mean corpuscular volume (MCV)	82	fL	83–101
Mean corpuscular hemoglobin (MCH)	27	pg	27–32
Mean corpuscular hemoglobin concentration (MCHC)	29	g/dL	31.5–34.5
Red cell distribution width (RDW)	27	%	11.6–14
Total leukocyte count	5.3	Thousand/µL	4–10
Neutrophil	60	%	40–80
Lymphocyte	35	%	20–40
Monocyte	5	%	2–10
Basophil	0	%	0–1
Eosinophil	0	%	1–6
Platelet count	3.2	Lakh/µL	150–410
Mean platelet volume	8.8	fL	6.8–10.9

1. **What are the probable reasons for anemia in the above mentioned patient?**
   Normocytic anemia

   The above mentioned patient is an elderly gentleman with multiple comorbidities with spinal tuberculosis.

   The CBC report is suggestive of normocytic hypochromic anemia.

   The differential diagnosis in this particular patient is as follows:
   - Dimorphic anemia (due to combined iron and vitamin B_{12} deficiencies)
   - Partially treated iron-deficiency anemia
   - Anemia due to renal disease
   - Anemia due to chronic inflammatory disease.

2. **What is the pathophysiology of anemia due to chronic disease states?**
   Hepcidin is the central molecule influencing iron metabolism in the body. As such, it plays an important role in pathophysiology of anemia due to chronic inflammatory states.

   Hepcidin is an acute-phase reactant protein, which physiologically controls the function of iron transporter ferroportin.

   Ferroportin is involved in intestinal absorption as well as release of iron from macrophages and the liver to the developed erythroid precursors in the bone marrow.

   In inflammatory states, high hepcidin levels downregulate ferroportin activity, resulting in suppressed erythropoiesis due to functional iron deficiency.[7]

3. **How do you differentiate iron deficiency anemia from anemia due to a chronic disease?**
   Anemia due to chronic disease is a diagnosis of exclusion in all cases.

   A thorough evaluation of all other possible causes of anemia is to be completed prior to this particular diagnosis.

   The biochemical picture of a patient with chronic disease can complicate the diagnosis of iron deficiency anemia as ferritin is an acute phase reactant.

   True or functional iron deficiency can be ascertained by a low transferrin saturation value. Elevated sTFR level and ratio of sTFR/log ferritin has been found to be more sensitive and specific for the diagnosis of iron deficiency anemia even in the presence of active infection.[8]

   Anemia associated with renal disease may also closely mimic anemia due to chronic disease. Approach to treatment remains common in these conditions. Addition of erythropoietin-stimulating agents (ESAs) after optimal correction of iron status leads to improvement in hemoglobin values.

   Note: Anemia due to chronic disease generally presents as mild-to-moderate anemia. The need for PRBC transfusion should trigger a thorough evaluation for alternate causes of drop in hemoglobin. For example, gastric bleed due to stress ulcers or drug-induced hemolysis.

4. **In which patients will you screen for a plasma cell dyscrasia?**
   Elderly patients presenting with unexplained anemia, especially if associated with back pain or decreased renal function, should be evaluated for plasma cell dyscrasia.

   Clues to the diagnosis are:
   - Presence of normocytic anemia
   - Raised total protein level with altered albumin:globulin ratio
   - Hypercalcemia and normal alkaline phosphatase levels

   These patients should be screened with a protein electrophoresis with immunofixation. Early referral to a hematologist is advisable to prevent pathological fractures and renal failure.

CASE SCENARIO 4: PANCYTOPENIA

You are asked to review an 18-year-old boy admitted with complaints of excessive fatigue since 3 months. He also complains of gum bleeding during brushing of teeth since 1 week. He was brought to the hospital with sudden onset of left-sided upper limb weakness and an episode of generalized tonic–clonic seizure.

He has no significant past history prior to this presentation.

His vital signs were as follows: Heart rate 64 beats/min, BP 170/100 mm Hg, RR 20 breaths/min, and SpO_2 100% on room air. His temperature was 37.4°C. He had severe pallor and multiple petechial spots on both arms and legs. He did not have hepatosplenomegaly.

Neuroimaging revealed a small intracerebral hematoma in right frontal region.

His CBC report was as follows:

		Units	Reference values
Hemoglobin	6.7	g/dL	13–17
Packed cell volume (hematocrit)	22	%	40–50
Red blood cell (RBC) count	3.1	Million/µL	4.5–5.5
Mean corpuscular volume (MCV)	88	fL	83–101
Mean corpuscular hemoglobin (MCH)	27	pg	27–32
Mean corpuscular hemoglobin concentration (MCHC)	29	g/dL	31.5–34.5
Red cell distribution width (RDW)	27	%	11.6–14
Total leukocyte count	1,800	Thousand/µL	4–10
Neutrophil	20	%	40–80
Lymphocyte	75	%	20–40
Monocyte	5	%	2–10
Basophil	0	%	0–1
Eosinophil	0	%	1–6
Platelet count	14,000	Lakh/µL	150–410
Mean platelet volume	9.2	fL	6.8–10.9

1. **How will you evaluate the above mentioned patient?**

    Pancytopenia

    The CBC report is suggestive of pancytopenia. Pancytopenia corresponds to a numerical reduction in all three cell lines—RBC, white blood cells (WBC), and platelets.

    A thorough history is imperative in narrowing the list of differential diagnoses in this condition. History related to recent infections, use of allopathic or alternative medicines, and recent history of jaundice is important to rule out reversible causes of pancytopenia. In any patient with pancytopenia, it is important to ascertain if bone marrow function is normal. Bone marrow function can be tested directly by the bone marrow aspiration and biopsy procedure or indirectly by testing for the reticulocyte count. A normal reticulocyte count may enable us to avoid a bone marrow biopsy procedure in patients with borderline cytopenia or in whom counts start to improve.

2. **How do you interpret the reticulocyte count?**
   Reticulocytes are the immediate precursors of the RBC. Reticulocyte count can serve as a reliable surrogate for bone marrow function.
   Reticulocytes are stained using the supravital staining methods using brilliant cresyl blue.
   To interpret the manual reticulocyte count, it needs to be corrected depending on the degree of anemia.
   - *Absolute reticulocyte count:* Retic (%) × RBC count
   - *Corrected reticulocyte count:* Reticulocyte count (%) × patient HCT/0.45
   - *Reticulocyte production index:* (Retic count (%)/maturation time) × (patient HCT/0.45)

   Normal HCT = 0.45
   Maturation time = Time taken for immature reticulocytes to be released into the blood (depends on degree of anemia)
   1 → HCT is 45
   1.5 → HCT is 35
   2 → HCT is 25
   2.5 → HCT is 20
   3 → HCT is <20.

3. **What are the differential diagnoses in a case of pancytopenia?**
   - Consumption disorders
   - Production disorders
   - Peripheral destruction and impaired production

4. **What is the role of a bone marrow biopsy in a patient with pancytopenia?**
   Bone marrow examination can be done from various sites such as:
   - Posterior superior iliac spine
   - Anterior superior iliac spine
   - Body of sternum
   - Anterior aspect of tibia (in very small children)

   Most commonly used site is the posterior superior iliac spine as it is superficial but sturdy and less frequently associated with procedural complications.
   Commonly used needle is the Jamshidi or hooked needle (11 × 10 Fr or 11 × 15 Fr).
   For pediatric patient, smaller needles, i.e., 13 × 10 Fr, is preferred.
   A variety of tests can be done from bone marrow samples depending on the indications for the biopsy.[9]

   Most commonly, morphological analysis is done:
   - **Bone marrow aspiration:** It is most important for cytological and morphological analysis of each marrow particles. It is very important for identification of normal erythropoiesis, myelopoiesis, and megakaryopoiesis. The identification of blasts, dysplasia, and infectious granulomas can be done from the bone marrow.[10]
   - **Bone marrow biopsy:** It gives a clearer picture regarding marrow cellularity and a panoramic view of the entire bone marrow. The presence of fibrosis, tuberculous granulomas, and megakaryocytes can be seen clearly in bone marrow biopsy blocks.

Special tests on bone marrow aspirate samples are as follows:
1. *Flow cytometry:* Specialized tests to identify hematological malignancies, immunodeficiencies, and paroxysmal nocturnal hemoglobinuria (PNH).
2. *Conventional karyotype:* It is important for diagnosis of chromosomal abnormalities like chronic myeloid leukemia and acute promyelocytic leukemia (APML). It is useful to prognosticate leukemia and myelodysplastic syndrome.
3. *Fluorescence in situ hybridization (FISH):* Quick and focused tests to identify commonly occurring genetic mutations in hematological conditions.
4. *Next-generation sequencing (NGS):* It is the State of the Art technique to identify mutations. This method is a revolutionary diagnostic and prognostic modality in various hematological malignancies.
5. *Bone marrow culture for bacterial/tuberculosis/fungal infection*—in cases with pyrexia of unknown origin.

CASE SCENARIO 5: MICROANGIOPATHIC HEMOLYTIC ANEMIA

You are asked to review a 24-year-old boy admitted with complaints of episodic memory loss and confusion since 10 days. He has a history of intermittent high grade fever spikes since 5 days. He also complains of spontaneous bruising over right arm developed 2 days back.

He was found to be in an unconscious state in the bathroom in the morning and rushed to the ER.

He has no significant past history prior to this presentation.

His vital signs were as follows: Heart rate 100 beats/min, BP 180/100 mm Hg, RR 18 breaths/min, and SpO$_2$ 100% on room air. His temperature was 39.1°C. He had pallor and a large ecchymotic patch over the right arm. He also had presence of wet purpura in the oral cavity. He did not have hepatosplenomegaly.

His CBC report was as follows:

		Units	Reference values
Hemoglobin	6.4	g/dL	13–17
Packed cell volume (hematocrit)	22	%	40–50
Red blood cell (RBC) count	2.9	Million/μL	4.5–5.5
Mean corpuscular volume (MCV)	98	fL	83–101
Mean corpuscular hemoglobin (MCH)	27	pg	27–32
Mean corpuscular hemoglobin concentration (MCHC)	29	g/dL	31.5–34.5
Red cell distribution width (RDW)	27	%	11.6–14
Total leukocyte count	12,500	Thousand/μL	4–10
Neutrophil	85	%	40–80
Lymphocyte	10	%	20–40
Monocyte	5	%	2–10

Contd...

Contd...

		Units	Reference values
Basophil	0	%	0–1
Eosinophil	0	%	1–6
Platelet count	22,000	Lakh/µL	150–410
Mean platelet volume	9.2	fL	6.8–10.9

1. **What is the differential diagnosis in the above mentioned patient?**

   Microangiopathic hemolytic anemia

   This patient has presented with a short history of neurological disturbance, fever spikes, and symptoms related to bleeding.

   The CBC report is suggestive of bicytopenia (anemia and thrombocytopenia).

   The differential diagnosis in this case would be:
   - Viral fever with encephalitis (probably dengue)
   - Thrombotic microangiopathy [thrombotic thrombocytopenic purpura (TTP)]
   - Acute leukemia with central nervous system (CNS) involvement
   - Disseminated tuberculosis.

2. **What are the causes of microangiopathic hemolytic anemia?**

   Thrombotic microangiopathy
   - With associated disease
   - TTP
   - Hemolysis, elevated liver enzymes, and low platelet count (HELLP)
   - Hemolytic–uremic syndrome (HUS).

3. **How do you evaluate a patient with suspected TTP?**

   Thrombotic thrombocytopenic purpura is a medical emergency. Any patient with suspected TTP should be managed in an ICU.

   The classical pentad of TTP is comprised of the following:
   - High-grade fever
   - Microangiopathic hemolytic anemia (MAHA)
   - Thrombocytopenia
   - Acute kidney injury
   - Neurological manifestations, including seizures or stroke

   All manifestations of the pentad may not be seen in every patient although some degree of thrombocytopenia is seen in all patients.

   The screening tests for TTP are:
   - Peripheral smear screening for schistocytes (>0.5% for every 1,000 RBCs counted)
   - LDH level [>upper limit of normal (ULN)]

   In any patient with significant schistocytes and raised LDH level, further tests and treatment should be planned on an urgent basis.

4. **What are the definitive tests to diagnose TTP?**
   Thrombotic thrombocytopenia purpura should be suspected in any patient with MAHA and thrombocytopenia.

   A quick evaluation to rule out disseminated intravascular coagulation (DIC), sepsis, autoimmune conditions, and malignancy should be done prior to initiation of plasma exchange.

   Bone marrow aspiration and biopsy to rule out an underlying hematological malignancy and an imaging study for solid organ malignancy should be done.

   Prior to initiation of plasma therapy, an ADAMTS13 level and an antibody to ADAMTS13 should be sent. An ADAMTS13 level <10% in an appropriate clinical setting is diagnostic of TTP. If antibody titer is significant, it indicates acquired TTP. In cases where antibody titer is negative, congenital TTP (Upshaw–Schulman syndrome) can be suspected.[11]

5. **How do you differentiate between TTP and HUS?**
   Hemolytic–uremic syndrome and TTP are both characterized as endotheliopathies—endothelial damage secondary to varied stimuli.

   Hemolytic–uremic syndrome is an endotheliopathy affecting the glomerular vessels, therefore presents with more severe acute kidney injury rather than thrombocytopenia.[12]

   Thrombotic thrombocytopenic purpura affects systemic capillaries, especially the vessels supplying the CNS, leading to neurological manifestations.

   Basic rule:
   If creatinine > 2.3 + platelet > 30,000 = HUS
   Creatinine < 2.3 + platelet < 30,000 = TTP

   A quick differentiation between these two conditions is important as plasma exchange is not successful in HUS.

REFERENCES

1. Whitehead RD Jr, Mei Z, Mapango C, Jefferds MED. Methods and analyzers for hemoglobin measurement in clinical laboratories and field settings. Ann N Y Acad Sci. 2019;1450(1):147-71.
2. Bain BJ, Bates I, Laffan MA (Eds). Dacie and Lewis Book of Practical Haematology, 12th edition. Elsevier; 2016.
3. Hoffman R, Benz EJ, Silberstein LE, Heslop HE, Weitz JI, Anastasi J, et al. (Eds). Hematology, 7th edition. Canada: Elsevier; 2018.
4. Green R. Vitamin B12 deficiency from the perspective of a practicing hematologist. Blood. 2017;129(19):2603-11.
5. Oberley MJ, Yang DT. Laboratory testing for cobalamin deficiency in megaloblastic anemia. Am J Hematol. 2013;88(6):522-6.
6. Torrez M, Chabot-Richards D, Babu D, Lockhart E, Foucar K. How I investigate acquired megaloblastic anemia. Int J Lab Hematol. 2022;44:236-47.
7. Fraenkel PG. Understanding anemia of chronic disease. Hematology Am Soc Hematol Educ Program 2015. 2015;1:14-8.
8. El-Gendy FM, El-Hawy MA, Rizk MS, El-Hefnawy SM, Mahmoud MZ. Value of Soluble Transferrin Receptors and sTfR/log Ferritin in the Diagnosis of Iron Deficiency Accompanied by Acute Infection. Indian J Hematol Blood Transfus. 2018;34(1):104-9.

9. Gnanaraj J, Parnes A, Francis CW, Go RS, Takemoto CM, Hashmi SK. Approach to pancytopenia: Diagnostic algorithm for clinical hematologists. Blood Rev. 2018;32(5):361-7.
10. Rindy LJ, Chambers AR. Bone Marrow Aspiration and Biopsy. In: StatPearls [Internet]. Treasure Island (FL): StatPearls Publishing; 2023.
11. Vesely SK, George JN, Lämmle B, Studt JD, Alberio L, El-Harake MA, et al. ADAMTS13 activity in thrombotic thrombocytopenic purpura-hemolytic uremic syndrome: Relation to presenting features and clinical outcomes in a prospective cohort of 142 patients. Blood. 2003;102(1):60-8.
12. Noris M, Remuzzi G. Hemolytic uremic syndrome. J Am Soc Nephrol. 2005;16(4):1035-50.

3.2: THROMBOCYTOPENIA

INTERPRETATION OF THE PLATELET COUNT
- The normal platelet count ranges from 150,000 to 400,000 cells/µL of blood.
- Thrombocytopenia is considered if platelet count is <100,000 cells/µL and thrombocytosis means a platelet count of >400,000 cells/µL—should be evaluated.

Approach to a Case of Thrombocytopenia/Thrombocytosis
Step 1: Peripheral smear examination
- Rule out pseudothrombocytopenia due to EDTA (ethylenediaminetetraacetic acid) induced agglutination/platelet satellitism—given as manual platelet count.
- Look at platelet morphology and size to rule out macrothrombocytopenia.
- Look at red blood cell (RBC) and white blood cell (WBC) morphology to identify clues to causes of thrombocytopenia.

Step 2:
- Get supplementary tests such as lactate dehydrogenase (LDH), serology, and liver function tests for further evaluation.
- Immature platelet fraction can be helpful in follow-up of cases where etiology is likely to be nonhematological.
- Ultrasound of the abdomen and pelvis should always be done to rule out chronic liver disease and organomegaly.
- In case of thrombocytosis, an iron profile and inflammatory markers should be sent to rule out cases with reactive thrombocytosis.

Step 3:
- Bone marrow biopsy should be done in cases with severe thrombocytopenia to rule out any abnormalities in the platelet precursor cells, i.e., megakaryocytes.
- In cases with immune thrombocytopenic purpura (ITP), bone marrow morphology will be normal.
- In case of suspected myeloproliferative neoplasm, bone marrow biopsy with mutation analysis will clinch the diagnosis.

Points to Remember
- Thrombocytopenia warrants evaluation only if platelet count is <100,000 cells/µL.
- Patients with thrombocytopenia should be treated with single donor platelets (SDPs) only if platelet count is <30,000 or if they have active ongoing bleeding.
- Most cases of mild thrombocytopenia may be due to pseudothrombocytopenia or macrothrombocytopenia—check manual platelet count before further evaluation.
- Mean platelet volume has clinical utility in hematology only in rare cases of suspected platelet function disorders with large platelets.
- Thrombocytosis is reactive in majority of cases with iron deficiency being a common reason—correction with intravenous (IV) iron reverses thrombocytosis.

BOX 1: Approach to thrombocytopenia.	
Confirm true thrombocytopenia	• If platelet clumps seen on smear, repeat blood draw in non-EDTA collection tube
Is the patient bleeding?	• Platelet goal >50 × 10^9 cells/L in non-CNS bleeding
Consider a TMA	• Evidence of hemolysis and schistocytes? – If yes, consider both primary and secondary TMA syndromes
Careful medication review	• Typical platelets fall 5–7 days after medication initiation • Inquire about heparin exposure within the past 100 days
Is the patient septic?	• Contributing cause in up to 75% of ICU patients
Consider hemodilution	• Common in the setting of massive transfusion
Are support devices contributing?	• Present in ≅25% of patients on VV-ECMO and 50% on IABP

(CNS: central nervous system; EDTA: ethylenediaminetetraacetic acid; IABP: intra-aortic balloon pump; ICU: intensive care unit; TMA: thrombotic microangiopathy; VV-ECMO: venovenous extracorporeal membrane oxygenation)

- Persistent thrombocytosis over 1 month in the absence of inflammatory etiology needs workup for myeloproliferative disorders **(Box 1)**.

CASE SCENARIO

A 46-year-old patient admitted in intensive care unit (ICU) for pulmonary embolism has his platelet count dropped to 40,000 on day 5 of hospital admission.

1. **What is the diagnosis?**

   Heparin-induced thrombocytopenic purpura

   Heparin-induced thrombocytopenia (HIT) is caused by platelet-activating immunoglobulin G (IgG) antibodies that bind to multimolecular complexes of platelet factor 4 (PF4) bound to heparin.

2. **Risk factors for heparin-induced thrombocytopenia**
   - *Heparin-type:* Unfractionated heparin (UFH) > low-molecular-weight heparin (LMWH) > fondaparinux
   - *Patient-type:* Postoperative > medical > pediatric/obstetric
   - *Dose:* Prophylactic dose > therapeutic dose > flushes
   - *Duration:* 11–14 days > 5–14 days > 4 days or less
   - *Sex:* Female > male

   Heparin-induced thrombocytopenia is relatively common, occurring in approximately 1–3% of postoperative patients and 0.2–0.5% of medical patients who receive UFH) derived from porcine intestine for 7–14 days.

3. **Differential diagnosis for heparin-induced thrombocytopenia**
   - Adenocarcinoma-associated disseminated intravascular coagulation (DIC)
   - Sepsis-associated microvascular thrombi
   - Septic emboli
   - Antiphospholipid antibody syndrome.

4. **Diagnosis of heparin-induced thrombocytopenia**

   Heparin-induced thrombocytopenia is a clinicopathological syndrome. Reports should be interpreted in the context of clinical symptoms.

   Assays for HIT antibodies can be classified as follows:
   - Platelet "activation" (functional) assays
   - PF4-polyanion "antigen" assays (immunoassays)

   Commonly available assays are immunoassays.

   In all patients with suspected HIT, pretest probability should be calculated prior to sending HIT antibody assay.

   Scoring system:
   - 1–3: Low risk of HIT
   - 4–5: Intermediate risk of HIT
   - 6–8: High risk of HIT

   Heparin-induced thrombocytopenia expert probability (HEP) scoring system can also be used to calculate pretest probability of HIT.

   A low 4T score despite HIT immunoassay positivity may not suggest clinically relevant HIT **(Table 1)**.

5. **Management of heparin-induced thrombocytopenia**
   - Assess clinically and radiologically for thrombosis (e.g., compression ultrasound for lower limb deep venous thrombosis).
   - Stop all heparin, including heparin flushes and possibly use of heparin-coated intravascular catheters (catheters left in situ for several days may not have much residual heparin).

TABLE 1: 4T scoring system.

4Ts category	2 points	1 point	0 point
Thrombocytopenia	Fall in platelet count >50% or platelet nadir ≥20,000	Fall in platelet count 30–50% or platelet nadir 10,000–19,000	Platelet count <30% or platelet nadir <10,000
Timing of platelet fall	Clear onset of thrombocytopenia 5–10 days after heparin exposure or sudden fall <1 day (prior heparin exposure within 30 days)	Probable onset of thrombocytopenia 5–10 days after heparin exposure or sudden fall <1 day (prior heparin exposure within 30–100 days)	Platelet fall <4 days after heparin exposure (no prior exposure)
Thrombosis or other sequelae	New thrombosis, skin necrosis, and acute systemic reaction post IV UFH bolus	Progressive or recurrent thrombosis, non-necrotizing skin lesions, and suspected thrombosis (not proven)	None
Other causes of thrombocytopenia	None apparent	Possible	Definite

(IV: intravenous; UFH: unfractionated heparin)

- Initiate treatment with an alternative anticoagulant, generally in therapeutic doses if HIT is strongly suspected (options—danaparoid, fondaparinux, lepirudin, argatroban, and bivalirudin).
- Although initial treatment decisions are made on clinical grounds, results of testing for HIT antibodies can influence subsequent treatment, including the decision to resume heparin if HIT has been ruled out.

Important Points to Remember
- Avoid platelet transfusions unless the patient is bleeding irrespective of platelet count.
- Avoid use of LMWH for management of HIT.
- To restart warfarin once platelet count is >150,000 and overlap with parenteral anticoagulant for at least 5 days.[1,2]

REFERENCES

1. Ostadi Z, Shadvar K, Sanaie S, Mahmoodpoor A, Saghaleini SH. Thrombocytopenia in the intensive care unit. Pak J Med Sci. 2019;35(1):282-7.
2. Greinacher A, Selleng S. How I evaluate and treat thrombocytopenia in the intensive care unit patient. Blood. 2016;128(26):3032-42.

3.3: INFECTION MARKERS AND THEIR INTERPRETATION

CASE SCENARIO

A 25-year-old female admitted in the intensive care unit (ICU) with severe urinary tract infection in septic shock.

Relevant blood investigations are:
- *Total count (TC):* 35,000
- *C-reactive protein (CRP):* 230
- *Procalcitonin (PCT):* 100

Kindly interpret the same.

Sepsis is a leading cause of mortality and morbidity and its early diagnosis is essential. Blood culture is the gold standard for the confirmation of bacteremia, but the delayed process of bacterial culture delays the diagnosis of sepsis; hence, the septic biomarkers come into play and help in diagnosis, assessing response to therapy, and prognosis on long-term basis.[1] Numerous biomarkers [interleukin 2 (IL-2) and IL-6 and tumor necrosis factor-α], leukotrienes, acute-phase proteins (CRP), PCT, and adhesion molecules have been evaluated with variable results, predicting the severity of sepsis and guiding its management.

INTERPRETATION OF WHITE BLOOD CELL COUNT

- The normal white blood cell (WBC) count ranges from 4,000 to 10,000 cells/μL of blood.
- Leukopenia means a total WBC count < 4,000 cells/μL and leukocytosis means a total WBC count of >10,000 cells/μL—should be evaluated.

Approach to a Case of Leukopenia/Leukocytosis

Step 1: Look at the differential WBC count. The normal differential count is:
- *Neutrophil:* 40–80%
- *Lymphocyte:* 30–40%
- *Monocyte:* 2–10%
- *Eosinophil:* 1–6%
- *Basophil:* 0–1%

Step 2: Peripheral smear examination
- Look for any abnormal cells in the peripheral smear examination.
- Toxic neutrophilic granules may indicate sepsis.
- Look at red blood cell (RBC) and platelet morphology.

Step 3: Get supplementary tests such as lactate dehydrogenase (LDH) and inflammatory markers for further evaluation.

Step 4: Consider bone marrow biopsy with flow cytometry if peripheral smear reveals presence of abnormal cells or in case of unexplained severe cytopenia.

Points to Remember
- Neutrophilic leukocytosis is most likely due to infectious/inflammatory etiology, likely due to a nonhematological condition.
- Neutropenia is an absolute neutrophil count <1,500 cells/μL and it should be evaluated urgently.
- Lymphocytosis in the setting of leukopenia may indicate viral infection.
- Eosinophil count >500 cells/μL is abnormal and >1,500 is considered to be hypereosinophilia.
- Significant basophilia in peripheral smear is abnormal and warrants further evaluation for chronic myeloid leukemia.
- Tuberculosis is an important cause of monocytosis in Indian population.

PROCALCITONIN

Procalcitonin is a 116-amino acid polypeptide precursor for the hormone calcitonin.

Procalcitonin has various immunologic functions, modulating the immune response during sepsis, infection, and inflammation including chemotactic functions.

Diagnosis of Infection and Sepsis

In the absence of other factors that may induce an increase in PCT levels, a PCT value of 0.25–0.5 ng/mL suggests the presence of a bacterial infection that requires antimicrobial treatment.

If PCT levels are <0.25 ng/mL, severe bacterial infection and sepsis are very unlikely; however, local infection may be present. The clinical relevance of the potential of PCT to differentiate between infectious and noninfectious causes of inflammation have been questioned in literature **(Table 1)**.

Noninfectious Causes of Procalcitonin Induction

Various causes of nonbacterial systemic inflammation and/or organ dysfunction that may be associated with elevated PCT levels include major surgery and trauma, severe burns, cardiogenic shock, and heat shock. Different types of immune therapies, such as granulocyte transfusions, administration of antilymphocyte globulin, anti-cluster of differentiation 3 (anti-CD3), or therapy with cytokines or related antibodies (alemtuzumab, IL-2, and tumor necrosis factor α) patients with acute graft-versus-host disease. Autoimmune diseases (Kawasaki disease and different types of vasculitis) and paraneoplastic syndromes.

TABLE 1: Procalcitonin values with category.

Procalcitonin (PCT) value (ng/mL)	Categories
<0.05	Healthy individuals
<0.5	Probability of sepsis is low and local infection is possible
0.5–2	Gray zone; recheck after 6–12 hours
>2	Probability of sepsis is high

TABLE 2: Guidelines for continuing or stopping antibiotics.

Concentration (μg/mL)	Interpretation
<0.25	Stopping of antibiotic strongly encouraged
Decrease by >80% from peak or concentration >0.25 but <0.5	Stopping of antibiotic encouraged
Decrease by <80% from peak or concentration >0.5	Continuing of antibiotic encouraged
Increase in concentration from peak or concentration >0.5	Changing of antibiotic strongly encouraged

Procalcitonin offers favorable kinetics, rising prior to 2 hours, reliably detectable between 2 and 4 hours, peaking at 6 hours, and maintaining a plateau through 8 and 24 hours. This response is considerably faster than that of CRP, whose levels increase slowly and only peak at 48 hours.

Also, PCT levels return to normal range faster than CRP, which makes it a better biomarker for sepsis.

A prospective study conducted by Patil et al.[2] revealed that the severity of sepsis was correlated with the proportionate increased level of serum PCT and CRP as well, with better correlation found between the PCT levels and APACHE II (Acute Physiology and Chronic Health Evaluation II) and Sequential Organ Failure Assessment (SOFA) scores. The parameters of sepsis, organ dysfunction, and mortality were significantly correlated with the serum PCT level.

However, a meta-analysis conducted by Sridharan et al.[3] concluded that the serum PCT concentrations have established utility in monitoring the clinical response to medical and surgical therapies for sepsis, and in surveillance for the development of sepsis in burns and ICU patients, and may have a role in guiding the de-escalation of antibiotic therapy. PCT does not appear to be affected by neutrophil count and has been evaluated in patients presenting with neutropenic fever. It was noted that PCT remains unaffected by corticosteroids when compared with CRP. PCT levels in candidemia do not appear to show the same level of elevation as in bacteremia. The sensitivity, specificity, and positive and negative predictive values for PCT were 100, 62, 57, and 100%, respectively.

The PRORATA (Procalcitonin to Reduce Antibiotic Treatments in Acutely ill patients) trial, a multicenter, prospective, open-label, and randomized control trial including 621 patients in eight ICUs in six hospitals found a 23% reduction in antibiotic usage on day 28; however, there was no difference in mortality.

Table 2 shows the guidelines for continuing or stopping antibiotics.

C-REACTIVE PROTEIN

C-reactive protein is an acute-phase reactant produced only by hepatocytes in response to inflammation or tissue injury. In healthy young adult volunteer blood donors, the median concentration of CRP is below 0.8 mg/L and can increase by 1,000-fold in response to an acute-phase stimulus.

C-reactive protein hepatic synthesis starts rapidly after a stimulus with rise noted by about 6 hours with peak around 48 hours and a plasma half-life of approximately 19 hours.

Elevated CRP levels in sepsis have been correlated with increased risk of death and organ failure, but in part due to the persistence of elevated levels were unable to predict survival when evaluating CRP trends.[2] CRP has been used successfully during initial sepsis diagnosis, but its specificity is further reduced later in the course due to persistently elevated levels.

Limitations of C-reactive Protein

- Delay in rise of CRP
- May increase during minor infections and do not adequately reflect the severity of the infection.
- May remain elevated for up to several days, even when infection is eliminated.
- Also elevated during inflammatory states.

REFERENCES

1. Nelson GE, Mave V, Gupta A. Biomarkers for sepsis: a review with special attention to India. Biomed Res Int. 2014:264351.
2. Patil H, Patil V. Comparative study of procalcitonin and C-reactive protein in patients with sepsis. J Nat Sci Biol Med. 2020;11(2):93.
3. Sridharan P, Chamberlain RS. The Efficacy of Procalcitonin as a Biomarker in the Management of Sepsis: Slaying Dragons or Tilting at Windmills? Surg Infect (Larchmt). 2013;14(6):489-511.

3.4: INTERPRETATION OF COAGULATION STUDIES

COAGULATION WORKUP

A screening coagulation workup includes a prothrombin time (PT), activated partial thromboplastin time (APTT), and a serum fibrinogen level.

Approach to a Case of Deranged Coagulation

Step 1: Reassessment of coagulation tests with a repeat sample with correct technique with optimal dilution of blood and 3.2% sodium citrate anticoagulant. Ratio of anticoagulant to blood is 1:9.

Step 2: In case of deranged PT-international normalized ratio (INR) and APTT both:
- Rule out liver disease with a liver function test (LFT) and ultrasound abdomen.
- Fibrinogen level should be seen to rule out disseminated intravascular coagulation.
- If both these conditions are ruled out, factor X deficiency and afibrinogenemia can be considered.
- Rarely combined deficiency of factors V and VIII may result in deranged PT-INR and APTT.
- In patients' polycythemia, appropriate correction for hematocrit should be made while collecting sample for coagulation studies.
  - For every mL blood collecting in a citrate tube, the amount of sodium citrate can be calculated by the following formula:

    Volume of citrate = 100 – hematocrit/595 – hematocrit
    × volume of anticoagulated blood in mL

Step 3: In case of isolated PT-INR derangement:
- A detailed bleeding history should be taken and ISTH bleeding assessment tool (BAT) score should be calculated.
- Rule out liver disease with LFTs and ultrasound of the abdomen.
- Do a mixing study—in case of full correction, run factor VII and IX levels.
- Combined factor VII/IX deficiency—vitamin K deficiency
- Isolated factor VII or IX deficiency require correction with appropriate factor therapy.
- If mixing study does not show 1:1 correction—indicates presence of a blocking antibody—refer to hematology for further evaluation.
- Cephalosporin exposure is associated with deranged PT-INR in the absence of coagulopathy.

Step 4: In case of isolated APTT derangement:
- A detailed bleeding history should be taken and ISTH BAT score should be calculated.
- Do a mixing study—in case of full correction, run factor VIII and IX levels.
- If mixing study does not show 1:1 correction—indicates presence of a blocking antibody—refer to hematology for further evaluation.
- In case factor VIII and IX levels are normal, factor XI and XII assessment should be done—especially if bleeding symptoms are absent.

1. **What are the effects of anticoagulants and how do I take this into account?**
   All anticoagulants [warfarin, heparins, and non-vitamin K antagonist oral anticoagulants (NOACs)] will increase the PT/INR and the APTT; this should, therefore, be considered when interpreting results. Patients on warfarin will have a specific target INR depending on the condition they have [atrial fibrillation (AF), valve replacements, etc.]; it is, therefore, a good idea to get a medical history from the patient.

   Antiplatelets, such as clopidogrel (P2Y12 inhibitor) and aspirin, will also cause derangement. These, however, will cause an increase in the overall bleeding time but will not affect PT or APTT.

2. **What key points should I take away from this?**
   Prothrombin time/International normalized ratio assesses the extrinsic pathway: Since factor VII pathology is rare, it is better used as a measure of overall clotting. It will, therefore, be affected in anticoagulant use, liver failure, and disseminated intravascular coagulation (DIC).

   Activated partial thromboplastin time assesses the intrinsic pathway: This, therefore, measures factors VIII [von Willebrand factor (vWF)], IX, and XI. The most common causes of increased APTT are hemophilia A (VIII), B (IX), C (XI), and possibly von Willebrand's disease (since vWF pairs with VIII).

   Bleeding time, although no longer used formally, measures the formation of the platelet plug. This will be affected by platelet disorders such as von Willebrand's disease (vWF), Bernard-Soulier syndrome glycoprotein Ib (GpIb), thrombotic thrombocytopenic purpura (TTP), immune thrombocytopenic purpura (ITP), hemolytic-uremic syndrome (HUS), and thrombocytopenia.

   Total clotting derangement is rare, but the cause must be identified quickly (e.g., DIC, malnutrition, or liver failure).

   Make sure to order complementary tests; full blood count (FBC) and LFTs can provide greater insight into a possible cause when correlated with the results of the coagulation screen.[1]

SPECIAL COAGULATION TESTS

Thromboelastography (TEG) is a viscoelastic hemostatic assay that measures the global viscoelastic properties of whole blood clot formation under low shear stress **(Fig. 1)**.
- TEG shows the interaction of platelets with the coagulation cascade (aggregation, clot strengthening, fibrin cross-linking, and fibrinolysis)
- It may or may not correlate with blood tests, such as INR, APTT, and platelet count (which are often poorer predictors of bleeding and thrombosis).

INDICATIONS

- Prediction of need for transfusion [maximum amplitude (MA) is a useful predictor in trauma].
- Guide transfusion strategy
- Liver transplantation, cardiac surgery, and trauma (to reduce transfusion requirement).

Case Scenarios and Interpretations of their Investigations

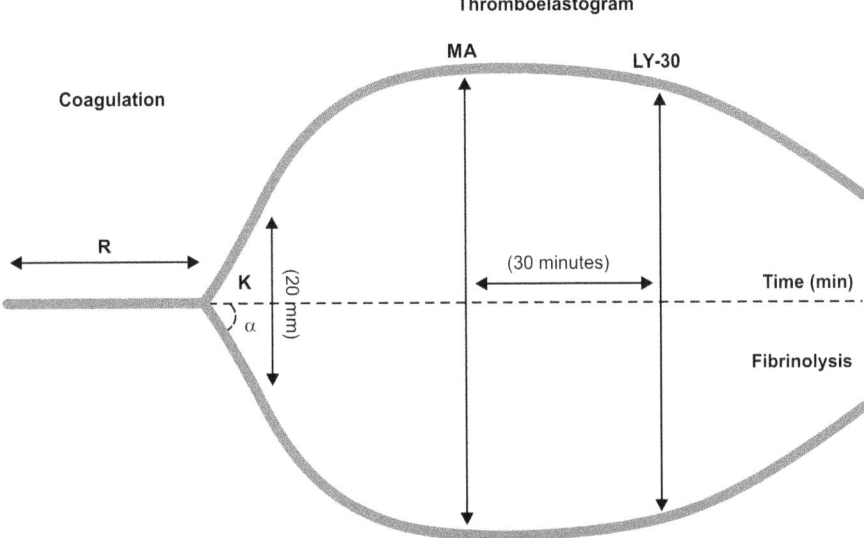

TEG	ROTEM	Description	Normal	Abnormality: Cause	Treatment
Reaction time (R valve)	Clotting time (CT)	Time till initiation of fibrin clot formation	5–10 minutes	↑ R value: ↓ factors	FFP protamine
K valve	Clot formation time (CFT)	Time to achieve 20 mm clot on assay representing thrombin-platelet interaction	1–5 minutes	↑ K/CFT value: ↓ fibrinogen	Cryoprecipitate fibrinogen
α-angle	α-angle	Rate at which fibrin cross-linking occurs	45–75°	↓ α angle: ↓ fibrinogen	Cryoprecipitate fibrinogen
Maximum amplitude (MA)	Maximum clot firmness (MCF)	Maximum strength of clot	50–75 mm	↓ MA/MCF: ↓ platelet count and/or function	Platelets DDAVP
LY-30	Clot lysis (CL)	Degradation of clot 30 minutes after MA/MCF	0–10%	↑ LY-30/CL: ↑ clot breakdoen	TXA Amicar

Fig. 1: Thromboelastogram interpretation. (DDAVP: deamino-8-D-arginine vasopressin; FFP: fresh frozen plasma; TEG: thromboelastography; TXA: tranexamic acid)

Specific parameters represent the three phases of the cell-based model of hemostasis: (1) initiation, (2) amplification, and (3) propagation:
- R value = Reaction time (s):
  - Time of latency from start of test to initial fibrin formation (amplitude of 2 mm)
  - Initiation phase
  - Dependent on clotting factors
- K = Kinetics (s):
  - Time taken to achieve a certain level of clot strength (amplitude of 20 mm)
  - Amplification phase
  - Dependent on fibrinogen
- Alpha = Angle (slope of line between R and K):
  - Measures the speed at which fibrin build up and cross-linking takes place; hence, assesses the rate of clot formation

Case Scenarios and Interpretations of their Investigations

- "Thrombin burst"/propagation phase
- Dependent on fibrinogen
- TMA = Time to maximum amplitude (s)
- MA = Maximum amplitude (mm):
  - Represents the ultimate strength of the fibrin clot, i.e., the overall stability of the clot
  - Dependent on platelets (80%) and fibrin (20%) interacting via GPIIb/IIIa
- A30 or LY30 = Amplitude at 30 minutes:
  - Percentage decrease in amplitude at 30 minutes post-MA
  - Fibrinolysis phase
- CLT = Clot lysis time (s)

Approximate normal values:
- *R:* 4–8 minutes
- *K:* 1–4 minutes
- α-*angle:* 47–74°
- *MA:* 55–73 mm
- *LY 30%:* 0–8%

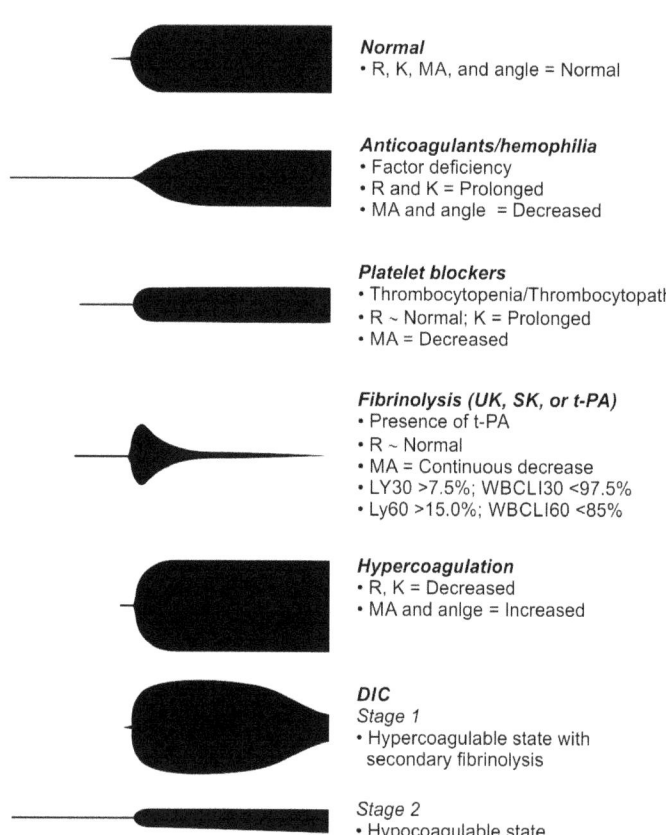

Normal
- R, K, MA, and angle = Normal

Anticoagulants/hemophilia
- Factor deficiency
- R and K = Prolonged
- MA and angle = Decreased

Platelet blockers
- Thrombocytopenia/Thrombocytopathy
- R ~ Normal; K = Prolonged
- MA = Decreased

Fibrinolysis (UK, SK, or t-PA)
- Presence of t-PA
- R ~ Normal
- MA = Continuous decrease
- LY30 >7.5%; WBCLI30 <97.5%
- Ly60 >15.0%; WBCLI60 <85%

Hypercoagulation
- R, K = Decreased
- MA and anlge = Increased

DIC
Stage 1
- Hypercoagulable state with secondary fibrinolysis

Stage 2
- Hypocoagulable state

(DIC: disseminated intravascular coagulation; K: kinetics; MA: maximum amplitude; R: reaction time; SK: streptokinase; t-PA: tissue plasminogen activator; UK: urokinase; WBCLI: whole blood clot lysis index)

THROMBOELASTOGRAPHY AS A GUIDE TO TREATMENT

- Increased R time → fresh frozen plasma (FFP)
- Decreased alpha angle → cryoprecipitate
- Decreased MA → platelets [consider DDAVP (deamino-8-D-arginine vasopressin)]
- Fibrinolysis → tranexamic acid (or aprotinin or aminocaproic acid).[2]

CASE SCENARIO

A 34-year-old male patient presented to the emergency room (ER) with three episodes of large hematemesis 2 hours back. On enquiry, his wife gives history of alcohol consumption. On examination, he is drowsy, incoherent, and disoriented. His pulse is 112 beats/min, blood pressure is 84/62 mm Hg, and oxygen saturation (SpO_2) is 94% on room air.

He is icteric with asterixis present. The abdomen is perturbant with flank fullness and shifting dullness is present with palpable spleen.

1. **How would you approach this patient of upper gastrointestinal (UGI) bleed?**

   Management

   It is evident from the history and clinical examination that he is suffering from chronic liver disease (CLD), and thus, variceal bleeding is the source of hematemesis.

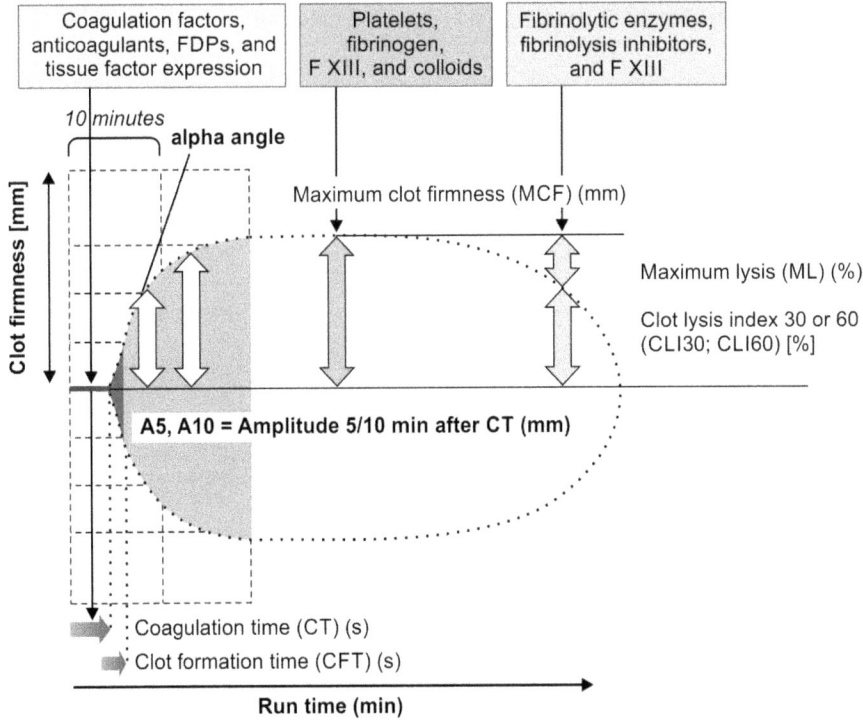

Fig. 2: Rotational thromboelastometry (ROTEM) graph.

He should be resuscitated as per C-A-B protocol and baseline investigation should be sent.

The initial tests (laboratory and imaging) include:
- *Anemia:* Hemoglobin may be normal in active bleeding and may take 6–24 hours to equilibrate. Other causes of anemia are common in cirrhotics. The liberal strategy of red blood cell (RBC) transfusion leads to worsening of portal hypertension in CLD patients.
- Thrombocytopenia is the most sensitive and specific laboratory parameter that correlates with portal hypertension and large esophageal varices.
- Elevated aspartate aminotransferase (AST), alanine aminotransferase (ALT), alkaline phosphatase, bilirubin, prolonged PT, and low albumin suggest cirrhosis.
- Blood urea nitrogen (BUN) is often elevated in gastrointestinal (GI) bleed.
- Sodium level may drop in patients treated with terlipressin.
- Coagulation profile
- Renal function
- Arterial blood gas
- Hepatitis serology
- TEG products to be given based on TEG.

Esophagogastroduodenoscopy should be done for diagnostic and therapeutic purposes. Hemoglobin should be checked 6–8 hourly and significant drop in hemoglobin should be considered as a sign of persistent bleeding or rebleeding. The patient can have persistent melena for 48–72 hours post episode of bleeding.[3,4]

REFERENCES

1. Hall JE (Ed). Guyton and Hall textbook of Medical Physiology, 13th edition. India: Saunders Elsevier; 2015.
2. Longmore M, Wilkinson IB, Baldwin A, Wallin E (Eds). Oxford Handbook of Clinical Medicine, 9th edition. India: Oxford University Press; 2014.
3. Le T, Bhushan V, Sochat M (Eds). First Aid for the USMLE Step 1 2019, 29th edition. McGraw-Hill Education; 2019.
4. Rang HP, Dale M, Flower RJ, Henderson G (Eds). Rang and Dale's Pharmacology, 8th edition. Churchill Livingstone; 2015.

3.5: RENAL FUNCTION TESTS URINE ANALYSIS

TESTS OF RENAL FUNCTION

Tests of renal function have utility in identifying the presence of renal disease, monitoring the response of kidneys to treatment, and determining the progression of renal disease.

Clinically, the most practical tests to assess renal function are to get an estimate of the glomerular filtration rate (GFR) and to check for proteinuria (albuminuria).

Creatinine

The most commonly used endogenous marker for the assessment of glomerular function is creatinine. The calculated clearance of creatinine is used to provide an indicator of GFR. Creatinine clearance is then calculated using the equation:

$$C = (U \times V)/P$$

where, C = clearance; U = urinary concentration; V = urinary flow rate (volume/time, i.e., mL/min), and P = plasma concentration

Creatinine clearance should be corrected for body surface area.

Creatinine is the by-product of creatine phosphate in muscle, and it is produced at a constant rate by the body. Creatinine is cleared from the blood entirely by the kidney. The amount of creatinine produced per day depends on muscle bulk, diet, and pregnancy. About 50% of kidney function must be lost before a rise in serum creatinine (SCr) can be detected. Thus, SCr is a late marker of acute kidney injury (AKI).

Blood Urea Nitrogen

About 85% of urea is eliminated via kidneys. Urea is increased earlier in renal disease.

The ratio of blood urea nitrogen (BUN): Creatinine can be useful to differentiate prerenal from renal causes when the BUN is increased. In prerenal disease, the ratio is close to 20:1, while in intrinsic renal disease, it is closer to 10:1. Upper gastrointestinal (GI) bleeding can be associated with a very high BUN to creatinine ratio (sometimes >30:1).

Cystatin C

Cystatin C is a low-molecular-weight protein, which is not affected by age, muscle bulk, or diet, and various reports have indicated that it is a more reliable marker of GFR than creatinine, particularly in early renal impairment.

TESTS OF TUBULAR FUNCTION

The renal tubules play a vital role in the reabsorption of electrolytes, water, and maintaining acid–base balance. Electrolytes—sodium, potassium, chloride, magnesium, and phosphate as well as glucose—can be measured in urine. Measurement of urine osmolality allows for assessment of concentrating ability of urine tubules. A urinary osmolality >750 mOsm/kg H_2O implies a normal concentrating ability of tubules. A water deprivation test can be used to exclude nephrogenic diabetes insipidus. Also, in distal renal tubular acidosis (RTA), an ammonium chloride test can be used to confirm the diagnosis of distal RTA with failure to acidify the urine to a pH of <5.3. In Fanconi's syndrome, there is aminoaciduria, glycosuria, phosphaturia, and bicarbonate wasting (proximal RTA).[1,2]

URINE ANALYSIS

Albuminuria refers to the abnormal presence of albumin in the urine. Urine albumin may be measured in 24-hour urine collections or early morning/random specimens as an albumin/creatinine ratio. The presence of albuminuria on two occasions with the exclusion of a urinary tract infection indicates glomerular dysfunction. The presence of albuminuria for three or more months is indicative of chronic kidney disease.

Frank proteinuria is defined as >300 mg/day of protein. Normal urine protein is up to 150 mg/day (30% albumin, 30% globulins, and 40% Tamm–Horsfall protein). In nephrotic syndrome, urine protein excretion exceeds 3.5 g/day and is associated with edema, hypoalbuminemia, and hypercholesterolemia. Cloudy urine may be seen in the presence of pyuria due to urinary tract infection. Nitrite and leukocyte esterase are indicators of urinary tract infection. Some bacteria, for example, *Enterobacteriaceae*, convert nitrates to nitrites.

Specific gravity is an indicator of the renal concentrating ability. Specific gravity is increased in concentrated urine and decreased in dilute urine.

Bilirubin is not detected in normal urine. Bilirubin is detected in the presence of conjugated hyperbilirubinemia.

Glucose is not detected in healthy patients but may be seen in diabetes mellitus, pregnancy, and renal glycosuria when the renal threshold of 180 mg/dL is decreased.

Blood may be present after renal tract injury or infection. Urine dipstick detects the globin portion of hemoglobin, and thus cannot detect the difference between the presence of myoglobin or hemoglobin in urine. In normal urine, red blood cell (RBC) per high-power field is between 0 and 3 and white blood cells (WBC) between 0 and 5.

Ketones are present in fasting, severe vomiting, and diabetic ketoacidosis. Urine dipstick only detects acetoacetate and acetone, not the ketone beta-hydroxybutyrate.

Urobilinogen may typically be present, but it is absent in conjugated hyperbilirubinemia and increased in the presence of prehepatic jaundice and hemolysis.

The microscopic analysis involves a wet-prep analysis of urine to assess the presence of cells, casts, and crystals as well as microorganisms. RBC casts usually denote glomerulonephritis, while WBC casts are consistent with pyelonephritis. The presence of WBC and WBC casts indicate infection, while RBC indicate renal injury, and RBC casts indicate tubular damage or glomerulonephritis. Hyaline casts consist of protein and may occur in glomerular disease. Fatty casts are seen in nephrotic syndrome. Crystals may also be identified in urine and are indicative of the following conditions:

- Triple phosphate crystals have the "coffin-lid" appearance and can be seen in alkaline urine and urinary tract infection.
- Uric acid crystals are needle shaped and are associated with gout.

- Oxalate crystals are envelope shaped and are present in ethylene glycol poisoning or primary and secondary hyperoxaluria.
- Cystine crystals are hexagonal and are observed in cystinuria.

The best specimen for urine analysis is a freshly voided midstream urine. Midstream urine is less likely to be contaminated by commensal bacteria and epithelial cells.

Fractional excretion of sodium (FeNa) is useful in distinguishing acute tubular necrosis (ATN) from prerenal uremia. Fractional excretion is calculated using the following formula:

$$FeNa = 100 \times (\text{urinary sodium} \times \text{serum creatinine})/(\text{serum sodium} \times \text{urinary creatinine})$$

A value <1% indicates a prerenal cause, and values > 2% indicate intrinsic causes. However, in patients receiving diuretic therapy, the FeNa is not reliable. Spot urine sodium concentrations of <20 mmol/L are an indicator of prerenal AKI. Fractional excretion of urea (FeUr) calculated similarly to FeNa using serum urea and urine urea instead of sodium can also be used to determine the presence of prerenal versus intrinsic AKI, with values <35% suggesting prerenal injury. A urine osmolality of >500 mOsm/kg is associated with prerenal causes, while an osmolality similar to serum (approximately 300 mOsm/kg) reflects an intrinsic cause.

NOVEL BIOMARKERS

New biomarkers include cystatin C, beta-2 microglobulin, retinol-binding protein, neutrophil gelatinase-associated lipocalin (NGAL), kidney injury molecule 1 (KIM-1), L-type fatty acid-binding protein (L-FABP), fibroblast growth factor 23 (FGF23), and beta-trace protein.

Urine Biochemical Analysis

Urine biochemical tests are easily available tests for any physician, but they are not frequently used in the intensive care setting. Acute renal dysfunction, use of diuretics, or intravenous (IV) fluid administration will alter urine test.

Urine spot test or 24-hour urine testing is still used in relatively stable patients to assess volume status (hypovolemia), dyselectrolytemia, and acid–base balance.

In critical care setting, spot urine testing is frequently used to assess urinary electrolytes, creatinine, urea, and osmolarity.

Can you outline the role of urine electrolytes in assessment of a critically ill patient?
Urinary sodium:
- Urinary sodium is used to assess hyponatremia and oliguria.
- It should be <20 mmol/L in hyponatremia and hypovolemia, which denotes appropriate sodium conservation.
- With hyponatremia, if urinary sodium is >40 mmol/L, it shows either urine wasting process [such as cerebral salt wasting, polyuric phase of ATN, and diuretics use] or urine is concentrated [syndrome of inappropriate antidiuretic hormone (SIADH)].

FeNa can be used to differentiate between prerenal and intrarenal causes of renal failure. It will be >2% in case of intrarenal causes of renal failure. Fractional excretion will be <1% for prerenal failure, which demonstrates the tendency to conserve sodium.

$$\text{Fractional excretion of sodium} = (\text{Urine sodium/serum sodium}) / (\text{urine creatinine/serum creatinine}) \times 100$$

Urine chloride:
- Urine chloride is used to investigate metabolic alkalosis.
- Urine chloride will be low (0–10 mmol/L) in cases of nonrenal causes of metabolic alkalosis, such as gastric loss and diuretics use.
- Urine chloride will be elevated (>20 mmol/L) whenever there will be inappropriate renal chloride loss because of corticosteroid excess, hypertension, or hyperaldosteronism.

Urine potassium:
- Urinary potassium should be low in case the patient is hypokalemic.
- High urinary potassium >15 mmol/L will be because of RTA (type I and II), hyperaldosteronism, corticosteroid excess, or diuretics use.
- Causes of low urinary potassium (<5–10 mmol/L) are diarrhea, laxative abuse, insulin, bicarbonate therapy, and hypokalemic periodic paralysis.

Urine anion gap:
- Used to assess normal anion gap metabolic acidosis to differentiate renal and gastrointestinal tract (GIT) causes of acidosis.[3,4]

$$\text{Urinary anion gap} = (UA - UC) = [Na^+] + [K^+] - [Cl^-]$$

- Urine anion gap is indirect assay of urine NH_4^+ excretion.
- In renal causes of normal anion gap acidosis, urine anion gap will be positive, while it will be negative for GIT causes of nonanion gap metabolic acidosis.

Urine osmolar gap:
- Urine osmolar gap calculation is used to diagnose causes of nonanion gap metabolic acidosis. It represents ammonium salt.

$$\text{Urine osmolar gap} = \text{Measured urine osmolality} - (2 \times Na + 2 \times K + urea/2.8)$$

- Urine osmolar gap/2 < 150 will present in RTA 1 and 4.
- If urine osmolar gap/2 > 400, look for GIT causes of nonanion gap metabolic acidosis.

How to diagnose prerenal failure with urine biochemistry?

Table 1 helps to differentiate between ATN and prerenal failure.

TABLE 1: A comparison of findings in prerenal and intrarenal failure.

	Intrarenal failure	Prerenal failure
Urine osmolality	<400–450 mOsm/kg	>450–500 mOsm/kg— concentrated urine is being passed
Urine sodium	High in acute tubular necrosis (ATN) (>40 mEq/L)	Low in prerenal disease (<20 mEq/L)
Urea/creatinine ratio	Normal in ATN	May be greater
Urine/serum creatinine ratio	>40	<20
Urine/serum osmolality	>1.0	>1.5
Fractional excretion of urea	>25%	<25%

Contd...

Contd...

	Intrarenal failure	Prerenal failure
Fractional excretion of sodium	>2%	<1%
Urine microscopy	ATN: • Muddy brown granular casts • Epithelial cell casts • Free epithelial cells	Nothing or hyaline casts (which are nonspecific)

CASE SCENARIO 1: AZOTEMIA

A 52-year-old unemployed male was admitted to a local hospital with severe fatigue and oliguria. On admission, he had been in bed for a month and could barely walk; also, at hospitalization, he was severely dehydrated, but was well circulated. Blood samples revealed extreme azotemia, hyperkalemia, metabolic acidosis, and anemia. Ultrasonography (USG) showed normal size kidneys without hydronephrosis. He received hemodialysis, blood transfusion, erythropoietin therapy, diuretics, and antihypertensive therapy. After 1 month, the patient was discharged. At this time, he was on hemodialysis three times a week.

Azotemia is a biochemical abnormality, defined as elevation or buildup of nitrogenous products (BUN—usually ranging from 7 to 21 mg/dL), creatinine in the blood, and other secondary waste products within the body. It is a typical feature of both acute and chronic kidney injury. There are three subtypes—prerenal, intrinsic, and postrenal azotemia.

Evaluation

When evaluating a patient for azotemia/AKI, there are many questions and physical findings that can help guide the appropriate diagnosis and treatment.
- *Evaluate volume status:*
  - Mucous membranes
  - Skin tenting
  - Edema (pitting/nonpitting)
  - Hepatojugular reflux
  - Pulmonary crackles
  - Ascites
- Check for signs of infection (lung, skin, and intra-abdominal), fever, chills, diaphoresis, cough, congestion, nausea, vomiting, diarrhea, dysuria, frequency, pyuria, and hematuria.

Prerenal findings: Sepsis/shock, burn, bleeding, dehydration (history of diarrhea and vomiting), skin tenting, worsening third spacing from intravascular depletion (pitting edema and ascites), and hypotension

Intrarenal findings: Nephrotoxic medication history, contrast exposure, poorly controlled hypertension, or diabetes mellitus

Postrenal findings: Flank pain, concerning for pyelonephritis; colicky pain, concerning for nephrolithiasis; boggy prostate, urinary hesitancy, and anuria, concerning for benign prostatic hyperplasia (BPH); smoking history, concerning for bladder cancer; and spinal cord trauma, concerning for neurogenic bladder.

Investigation?

Laboratory evaluation for azotemia includes a basic metabolic panel (BMP), BUN/creatinine, urinary sodium (Na), protein, creatinine, urea, urine osmolality, and urinalysis (UA). Radiographic evaluation can be with a renal USG, computed tomography (CT) of the abdomen and pelvis with or without contrast, or renal Doppler examination.

Diagnosis of azotemia can be made by a BUN > 21 mg/dL.

Significant findings for prerenal azotemia are as follows:
- *BUN:* Creatinine ratio > 20:1
- FeNa < 1 and FeUr < 35%
- Urine osmolality 500 mOsm/kg
- UA can show hyaline casts.

Intrarenal Azotemia
- *BUN*: Creatinine ratio < 20:1
- FeNa > 2 and FeUr > 50%
- Urine osmolality < 300 mOsm/kg
- *UA*: Cellular debris, muddy brown casts red cell casts, eosinophils, + proteinuria.

Postrenal Azotemia
- *BUN*: Creatinine ratio < 20:1
- FeNa > 2
- Urine osmolarity < 300 mOsm/kg
- *UA*: WBC casts
- *Imaging findings*: Pyelonephritis, nephrolithiasis, and bladder mass.
Treatment will be according to the cause of the same.

Differential Diagnosis
Differentials for an elevated BUN (azotemia) are:
- GI bleeding
- Corticosteroid use
- Ketoacidosis
- States of protein catabolism
- Congestive heart failure (CHF)
- Hyperalimentation [total parenteral nutrition (TPN)].[5]

CASE SCENARIO 2: NEPHROTIC SYNDROME

A 48-year-old male with no comorbidities or major illness in the past was admitted with chief complaints of facial puffiness developed since 7–10 days, more in morning time, and passing turbid urine for almost 1 week. Facial puffiness was present, which initially started as periorbital edema. Urine output was decreased He had bilateral lower limb swelling since 7 days.

General examination revealed pallor + blood pressure of 140/90 mm Hg.

Urine biochemistry revealed protein 3^+, RBC 30–40, and blood urea was raised to 500 µmol/L and USG showed bilateral mildly enlarged kidneys.

1. **What are the differential diagnosis as per history?**
   Nephrotic syndrome (NS): It is a clinical syndrome defined by massive proteinuria (>40 mg/m^2/h) responsible for hypoalbuminemia (<30 g/L), with resulting hyperlipidemia and edema.

2. **What investigations should be sent?**
   Urine tests: Nephrotic-range proteinuria will be apparent by 3$^+$ or 4$^+$ readings on the dipstick, which correlates with a daily loss of 3 g or more, and thus is in the nephrotic range. Urine samples collected over a 24-hour period (for an accurate measure), proteinuria (3 g protein) is diagnostic.
   Urinalysis may demonstrate casts (hyaline, granular, fatty, waxy, or epithelial cell).
   Lipiduria, the presence of free lipid or lipid within tubular cells, within casts, or as free globules, suggests a glomerular disorder.
   Blood tests: The serum albumin level is classically low in nephrotic syndrome and often is <2.5 g/dL. Creatinine concentrations vary by degree of renal impairment. Total cholesterol and triglyceride levels are typically increased.
   Test results may alter management and preclude the need for biopsy.
   Ultrasonography and renal biopsy may be needed as added investigations.

3. **What are the primary as well secondary causes?**
   - *Primary causes:* These are minimal-change nephropathy, focal glomerulosclerosis, membranous nephropathy, and hereditary nephropathies.
   - *Secondary causes:* These include diabetes mellitus, immune disorder, and infection.

4. **What are the stages?**
   - *Remission:* Urine albumin nil or trace for three consecutive early morning specimens
   - *Relapse:* Urine albumin 3$^+$ or 4$^+$ (or proteinuria >40 mg/m^2/h) for three consecutive early morning specimens, having been in remission previously.
   - *Frequent relapses:* Two or more relapses in the initial 6 months or more than four relapses in any 12 months.
   - *Steroid dependence:* Two consecutive relapses when on alternate day steroids or within 14 days of its discontinuation.
   - *Steroid resistance:* Absence of remission despite therapy with daily prednisolone at a dose of 2 mg/kg/day for 4 weeks.
   - *Congenital:* Presenting within the first 3 months of life, and in these children, there is usually a genetic mutation.[6]

CASE SCENARIO 3: RENAL TUBULAR ACIDOSIS

A 26-year-old-male mechanic brought to the emergency department (ED) with overdose of unknown substance.
Vitals are as: Heart rate (HR) 100 beats/min, blood pressure 80/50 mm Hg, Glasgow Coma Scale (GCS) 12/15, oxygen saturation (SpO$_2$) 100% on room air, and respiratory rate (RR) 34 breaths/min.

		Reference values
pH	7.15	7.35–7.45
PaO$_2$ (mm Hg)	111	83–108
PaCO$_2$ (mm Hg)	20	32–48
HCO$_3^-$ (mmol/L)	8	22–28
Glucose (mg/dL)		65–95
Lactate (mmol/L)	5.2	0.4–0.8
Sodium (mmol/L)	135	136–145
Potassium (mmol/L)	5.5	3.4–4.5
Chloride (mmol/L)	96	98–107
Creatinine (mg/dL)	2.5	0.45–1.09

1. **What are the different types of RTA?**

   Subtypes

   The subtypes are as follows:
   - *Type 1:* Distal RTA
   - *Type 2:* Proximal RTA
   - *Type 3:* Mixed RTA

2. **How will you evaluate RTA?**

   Evaluation

   Plasma HCO$_3$ levels:
   - *Type 1:* <10–20 mEq
   - *Type 2:* 12–18 mEq/L
   - *Type 4:* >17 mEq/L

   Plasma potassium: Low in type 1 and 2 and high in type 4 and 1.

   BUN/Creatinine: Normal or near normal (rules out renal failure as the cause of acidosis).

   UA: Urine pH inappropriately alkaline (>5.5) despite metabolic acidosis in type 1, also in type 2, if HCO$_3$ above reabsorptive threshold (12–18 mEq/L), and acidic <5.5 in type 2 and 4.

   Urine culture: Rule out urinary tract infection with the urea-splitting organism as it may elevate urine pH.

   Urine anion gap [(Na + K) – Cl]: Positive gap signifies low NH$_4$Cl excretion, which causes decreased chloride in urine along with hyperchloremic metabolic acidosis, suggesting RTA.

   Specific Tests

   Bicarbonate infusion test: Fractional bicarbonate excretion is measured after an infusion of bicarbonate. The serum bicarbonate concentration approaches the normal level in the body after the infusion, which is more than the reabsorption threshold of the patient with type 2 proximal RTA. Urine pH rises because of the appearance of >15% of filtered bicarbonate in urine.

   Urine Na: Type 4 RTA presents with persistently high urine Na despite restricted Na diet because of aldosterone deficiency or resistance.

Treatment

Correction of chronic academia with alkali administration is warranted to prevent its catabolic effects on bone and muscles. Most of the bicarbonate is absorbed in the proximal tubule, so distal RTA is relatively easy to correct. Proximal tubule will absorb the given bicarbonate and correct acidosis.

High doses of bicarbonate >10 mmol/kg/day are required to treat type 2 RTA. Increased bicarbonate concentration in urine induced by alkali therapy also increases urinary potassium losses because increased sodium and water delivery to the distal tubule stimulate potassium secretion. Thiazide diuretics cause volume depletion, which will enhance bicarbonate reabsorption in type 2 RTA.

Hypophosphatemia due to decreased proximal phosphate reabsorption and reduced activation of vitamin D also occurs in some patients and may be a major contributor to the development of bone disease. Thus, both phosphate and vitamin D supplementation may be required to normalize the serum phosphate and reverse the metabolic bone disease.

Fludrocortisone 0.1 mg/day is effective in managing hyperkalemia associated with aldosterone deficiency. However, it is not usually used because hypertension, heart failure, and edema may be exacerbated in patients with renal insufficiency.[7]

CASE SCENARIO 4: POSTOBSTRUCTIVE DIURESIS

A 65-year-old patient presented to the ED with sudden anuria. The patient also complained of decreasing urine output and interrupted urine since 7 days and loin pain over the right side. The patient is a farmer by occupation; USG showed calculi in the right and left ureters, with bilateral hydronephrosis. The patient was taken for surgery and bilateral double J (DJ) stenting was done and the patient started pouring 500 mL urine hourly postoperative.

Postobstructive diuresis is an abnormal condition of prolonged polyuria, involving both excessive salt and water loss, after the acute drainage and decompression of a distended bladder, typically from urinary retention.

Normal maximum bladder capacity is about 450–500 cc. Postobstructive diuresis is not typically an issue unless the residual urine is 1,500 cc or more.

By definition, postobstructive diuresis is the condition of prolonged urine production of at least 200 cc for at least two consecutive hours immediately following the relief of urinary retention or similar obstructive uropathy. It may also be defined as >3,000 cc over 24 hours.

Management

Urine output should be monitored at least every 2 hours. Serum electrolytes including sodium, potassium, urea, creatinine, magnesium, and phosphate should be checked every 12 hours initially. They are allowed unrestricted access to water for drinking. Daily weights are helpful. Urine samples can be collected for urinary measurements of osmolality, sodium, and potassium.

Random urine sodium levels >40 mEq/L are suggestive of possible renal tubular injury, which can progress to pathologic postobstructive diuresis.

Intravenous fluid support should be normal saline and limited to no >75% of the prior 1–2-hour urine production to avoid stimulation of further diuresis.

Pathological postobstructive diuresis puts the patient at risk for hypovolemia and hemodynamic instability as well as acid–base disturbances and electrolyte imbalances. Careful monitoring of fluid status, weight, serum electrolytes, and renal function is necessary to minimize the duration of the condition and facilitate recovery.[8]

CASE SCENARIO 5: RHABDOMYOLYSIS

A 21-year-old man had bilateral lower limb pain and soreness and dark brown urine after lower extremity training. Laboratory results showed that creatine kinase (CK) and myoglobin increased to 140–500 IU/L and 8,632 µg/L, respectively, with elevated liver enzymes, SCr, and proteinuria.

1. **What is your diagnosis? How will you evaluate?**
   Rhabdomyolysis is the breakdown of skeletal muscle fibers with leakage of potentially toxic intracellular contents into the systemic circulation, characterized by elevated plasma CK, myoglobinuria, and risk of renal impairment.

   Causes
   The causes can be traumatic or nontraumatic.

   Traumatic causes:
   - Victims of polytrauma are prone to crush syndrome and may develop severe compartment syndrome[9]
   - Prolonged immobilization due to coma, intoxication with alcohol and opiates, hip fracture, and surgeries
   - Fractures of lower extremities (tibial fracture), arterial occlusion from prolonged immobilization, tourniquet, and surgical clamping
   - Strenuous muscular exercise, especially in untrained individuals, status epilepticus, delirium tremors, phencyclidine overdose, tetanus, and rarely sepsis.

   Nontraumatic or nonphysical causes:
   - *Medications:* Alcohol, colchicine, carbon monoxide, statins, and illicit drug use.[10]
   - *Infections:* Pyomyositis [MRSA (methicillin-resistant *Staphylococcus aureus*)], septic shock, and toxic shock syndrome
   - *Electrolyte abnormalities:* Hypokalemia, hypophosphatemia, hyperosmolar conditions, hypo- and hypercalcemia, and severe dehydration
   - *Endocrine:* Hyperosmolar hyperglycemic state, severe diabetic acidosis with coma, and myxedema
   - *Myopathies:* Insect bite and snake venom and carbon monoxide
   - *Autoimmune myositis:* Polymyositis and dermatomyositis
     - *Hemoglobinopathy:* Sickle-cell trait.
     - *Dysregulated body temperature:* Neuroleptic malignant syndrome, malignant hyperthermia (inhaled anesthetic agents with or without succinylcholine), near drowning, hypothermia, and frostbite

2. **What is the triad of rhabdomyolysis?**
   Rhabdomyolysis clinically is a triad of myalgia, myoglobinuria (tea-colored urine), and weakness.

Pathophysiology

Mechanisms of renal failure due to rhabdomyolysis are as follows:
- Renal vasoconstriction
- Intraluminal cast formation
- Direct heme-protein-induced cytotoxicity

Complications of rhabdomyolysis are as follows:
- Hyperkalemia (early)
- Hypocalcemia (secondary to increased phosphate)
- Myoglobin release leading to acute renal failure (late)
- Disseminated intravascular coagulation (DIC) due to release of thromboplastins (rare)
- Shock due to "third space" losses from extravasation of fluid from extensively damaged muscle (if severe).

3. **How to evaluate a patient with rhabdomyolysis?**
   - The hallmark of acute rhabdomyolysis is elevated CPK levels. In addition, reddish-brown urine from myoglobinuria may be present in 50% of cases. Normal CPK levels are 20–200 IU/L. Elevated levels usually at least five times the upper limit of normal are considered rhabdomyolysis. Its half-life is 36 hours. Serum CPK levels begin to rise within 2–12 hours after the injury peaks within 1–5 days. It declines after 3–5 days in the absence of muscle injury. Suspect continued muscle injury and compartment syndrome in cases of persistently elevated CPK levels.
   - With the release of an excess amount of myoglobin, heme-containing myoglobin is excreted in urine resulting in tea-colored urine. Its half-life is about 2–4 hours and is metabolized into bilirubin. Myoglobinemia can be detected before the elevation of CPK. Because of the shorter half-life and rapid metabolism, myoglobinuria may not always be detected. Urine dipstick detects hemoglobin and myoglobin as blood; a follow-up microscopic evaluation for RBC should be done to rule out hemoglobinuria. The sensitivity of myoglobinuria in rhabdomyolysis is <25%.
   - Hyperkalemia
   - Hypocalcemia
   - Increased uric acid
   - Metabolic acidosis with or without anion gap
   - Electrocardiogram (ECG) may show peaked T waves, prolonged PR interval, wide QRS interval with or without conduction blocks, ventricular tachycardia, and asystole secondary to hyperkalemia. Hypocalcemia can manifest as QTC prolongation.

The causes of AKI are as follows:
- Hypovolemia
- Drugs
- Dehydration
- Hypoperfusion
- Pigment-induced distal tubular damage

Acute kidney injury is the most common complication of rhabdomyolysis. Patients with CK levels of >40,000 IU/L have an increased risk of AKI.

Disseminated intravascular coagulation is another dreadful complication. Also, look for compartment syndrome.

Investigation
- ECG (hyperkalemia and hypocalcemia)
- Blood gas (hyperkalemia and metabolic acidosis)
- Elevated CPK—peaks <24 hour, then decreases by ~40% per day after the initial insult. If >5,000, there is 50% chance of AKI; persistent or increasing CK suggests ongoing cause/precipitant or development of a compartment syndrome)
- Complete blood count
- Urine routine
- Coagulation profile
- Urine myoglobin (dipstick may indicate presence of blood)
- Hyperkalemia
- Renal failure from myoglobinuria
- Metabolic acidosis
- Hyperphosphatemia
- Hypokalemia
- Hyperuricemia

3. **What is the role of urine alkalinization?**

Alkalinization of urine is done to prevent precipitation of myoglobin in the distal convoluted tubule. The goal of alkaline fluid infusion is to maintain a serum pH not to exceed 7.5 and a urine pH just above 6.5. Prompt discontinuation of bicarbonate in IV fluids should be done when serum pH is at 7.5.[5,6]

REFERENCES

1. Reddi AS (Ed). Interpretation of Urine Electrolytes and Osmolality. Fluid, Electrolyte, and Acid - Base Disorders. New York: Springer; 2014. pp. 13-9.
2. Harrington JT, Jordan JC. Measurement of urinary electrolytes --indications and limitations. N Engl J Med. 1975;293(24):1241-3.
3. Kirschbaum B, Sica D, Anderson FP. Urine electrolytes and the urine anion and osmolar gaps. J Lab Clin Med. 1999;133(6):597-604.
4. Cadogan M. (2023). Urine Electrolytes. [online] Available from: https://litfl.com/urine-electrolytes/ [Last accessed August, 2023].
5. Tyagi A, Aeddula NR. Azotemia. [Updated 2023 May 14]. In: StatPearls [Internet]. Treasure Island (FL): StatPearls Publishing; 2023 Jan. Available from: https://www.ncbi.nlm.nih.gov/books/NBK538145/.
6. Lu H, Xiao L, Song M, Liu X, Wang F. Acute kidney injury in patients with primary nephrotic syndrome: influencing factors and coping strategies. BMC Nephrol. 2022;23(1):90.
7. Firth JD, Sayer JA, Karet FE. The renal tubular acidosis. In: Firth JD, Conlon C, Cox T (Eds). Oxford Textbook of Medicine, 6th edition (Oxford, 2020; online edn, Oxford Academic, 1 Jan. 2020), https://doi.org/10.1093/med/9780198746690.003.0505.
8. Leslie SW, Sajjad H, Sharma S. Postobstructive Diuresis. [Updated 2022 Nov 28]. In: StatPearls [Internet]. Treasure Island (FL): StatPearls Publishing; 2023 Jan. Available from: https://www.ncbi.nlm.nih.gov/books/NBK459387/.
9. Coban YK. Rhabdomyolysis, compartment syndrome, and thermal injury. World J Crit Care Med. 2014;3(1):1-7.
10. Hohenegger M. Drug-induced rhabdomyolysis. Curr Opin Pharmacol. 2012;12(3):335-9.

3.6: LIVER FUNCTION TESTS

INTRODUCTION

The term "liver function tests" is a misnomer as many of the tests do not comment on the function of the liver, but rather pinpoint the source of the damage. Elevations in alanine transaminase (ALT) and aspartate aminotransferase (AST) out of proportion to alkaline phosphatase (ALP), and bilirubin denote a hepatocellular disease. An elevation in ALP and bilirubin in disproportion to ALT and AST would characterize a cholestatic pattern. A mixed injury pattern is defined as an elevation of ALP and AST/ALT levels. Isolated hyperbilirubinemia is defined as an elevation of bilirubin with normal ALP and AST/ALT levels.

The R ratio has been used to assess whether the pattern of liver injury is hepatocellular, cholestatic, or mixed. The R ratio is calculated by the formula R = [ALT value ÷ ALT upper limit of normal (ULN)] ÷ (ALP value ÷ ALP ULN). An R ratio of >5 is defined as hepatocellular, <2 is cholestatic, and 2–5 is a mixed pattern.

The actual function of the liver can be graded based on its ability to produce albumin as well as vitamin K-dependent clotting factors.

A borderline AST and/or ALT elevation is defined as <2× ULN, a mild AST and/or ALT elevation as 2–5× ULN, moderate AST and/or ALT elevation 5–15× ULN, severe AST and/or ALT elevation >15× ULN, and massive AST and/or ALT >10,000 IU/L.

DIFFERENTIAL DIAGNOSIS BASED ON ELEVATED LIVER FUNCTION TESTS

Hepatocellular pattern: Elevated aminotransferases out of proportion to ALP
- *ALT-predominant:* Acute or chronic viral hepatitis, steatohepatitis, acute Budd–Chiari syndrome, ischemic hepatitis, autoimmune, hemochromatosis, medications/toxins, autoimmune, alpha-1-antitrypsin deficiency, Wilson disease, and celiac disease
- *AST-predominant:* Alcohol related, steatohepatitis, cirrhosis, and nonhepatic (hemolysis, myopathy, thyroid disease, and exercise)

Cholestatic pattern: Elevated ALP + gamma-glutamyl transferase (GGT) + bilirubin out of proportion to AST and ALT
- *Hepatobiliary causes:* These are bile duct obstruction, primary biliary cirrhosis, primary sclerosing cholangitis, medication induced, infiltrating diseases of the liver (sarcoidosis, amyloidosis, and lymphoma among others), cystic fibrosis, hepatic metastasis, or cholestasis.
- *Nonhepatic causes:* These are bone disease, pregnancy, chronic renal failure, lymphoma or other malignancies, congestive heart failure, childhood growth, infection, or inflammation.

COMPONENTS OF LIVER FUNCTION TEST

Hepatocellular Laboratories

Aminotransferase includes AST and ALT. They are markers of hepatocellular injury. AST is present as cytosolic and mitochondrial isoenzymes and is found in the liver, cardiac muscle, skeletal muscle, kidneys, brain, pancreas, lungs, leucocytes, and red cells. It is not as sensitive or specific for the liver as ALT.

Alanine transaminase is a cytosolic enzyme that is found in high concentrations in the liver. The half-life of ALT is approximately 47 ± 10 hours. ALT is usually higher than AST in most types of liver disease in which the activity of both enzymes is predominantly from the hepatocyte cytosol.

Cholestasis Laboratories

Alkaline phosphatase is part of a family of zinc metalloenzymes that are highly concentrated in the microvilli of the bile canaliculus as well as several other tissues (e.g., bone, intestines, and placenta).

Glycoprotein GGT is more specific than ALP as it is not present in bone.

Markedly increased lactate dehydrogenase (LDH) levels are observed in hepatocellular necrosis, shock liver, lymphoma, or hemolysis associated with liver disease.

Bilirubin is the end product of heme catabolism, with 80% derived from hemoglobin. Unconjugated bilirubin is transported to the liver loosely bound to albumin.

Synthetic Function Tests

- Albumin is synthesized by the hepatic parenchymal cells. With any liver disease, there is a fall in serum albumin, reflecting decreased synthesis. If liver function is normal and serum albumin is low, this may reflect poor protein intake (malnutrition) or protein loss (nephrotic syndrome, malabsorption, or protein-losing enteropathy).
- Except for factor VIII, all other coagulation factors are synthesized by the liver. Suppose the synthetic function of the liver is normal and prothrombin time is delayed. This may indicate treatment with warfarin, consumptive coagulopathy (e.g., disseminated intravascular coagulopathy), or vitamin K deficiency.

Alcoholic Liver Disease

In patients with alcohol use disorder, AST to ALT ratio is generally at least 2:1, which shows a high level of AST activity in alcoholic liver disease. Elevated GGT, along with AST, also suggests alcohol abuse. GGT should not be used alone since it is not very specific for alcohol.[1]

CASE SCENARIO 1: ACUTE ON CHRONIC LIVER FAILURE

A 54-year-old lady, a known case of hypothyroidism for 12 years on thyroxine supplementation, presented with fatigue for 3 months and pruritus for 2 months, which was initially mild, but now progressed to severe and disturbing her sleep. She also noticed mild-yellowish discoloration of her eyes for 1 month. On examination, she has icterus, rest all vitals were within normal limits.

1. **How to approach for investigation and treatment for this patient?**
   Diagnosis
   Cholestasis means stagnation (stasis) of bile (chole). The cholestatic disorder of liver is due to either production, delivery, or recycling of the bile.

TABLE 1: Features of cholestasis.		
Features	Extrahepatic	Intrahepatic
Abdominal pain	+	–
Fever	+	–
History of previous hepatobiliary surgery	+	–
History of prodrome	–	+
History of drug intake	–	+
Sepsis	–	+
Family history	–	+

Broadly, cholestasis disorders of the liver are divided into intrahepatic causes or extrahepatic causes.

2. **How do we evaluate cholestasis?**
   There are few points on the history taking, which can differentiate between extrahepatic or intrahepatic cause of cholestasis **(Table 1)**.
   In this patient, as there is absence of abdominal pain and no history of any previous surgery and there is presence of history of hypothyroidism, which is an autoimmune disorder, it is likely to be an intrahepatic cause of cholestasis.

3. **What are the various causes of intrahepatic cholestasis and which investigations should be done for the same?**
   - *Drug-induced:* History of precedent drug intake (commonly used antibiotics such as azithromycin, amoxicillin–clavulanate, antitubercular drugs, etc.) or history of complementary and alternative medication (CAM) intake.
   - *Cholestatic phase of viral hepatitis such as hepatitis A or hepatitis B:* Serum hepatitis A virus (HAV) immunoglobulin M (IgM) and IgG, hepatitis B surface antigen (HbsAg), and hepatitis B core antibody.
   - *Autoimmune hepatitis:* Antinuclear antibody (ANA), anti-smooth muscle antibody (ASMA), anti–liver–kidney microsome type 1 (anti–LKM-1) antibody, and serum IgG level.
   - *Primary biliary cholangitis (PBC):* Antimitochondrial antibody (AMA) level
   - *Primary sclerosing cholangitis (PSC):* Perinuclear antineutrophil cytoplasmic antibody (p-ANCA) and magnetic resonance cholangiopancreatography (MRCP)
   - *Intrahepatic cholestasis of pregnancy (ICP):* Serum bile acid level
   - Total parenteral nutrition- (TPN)-induced cholestasis
   - *Progressive familial intrahepatic cholestasis (PFIC) and benign recurrent intrahepatic cholestasis (BRIC):* Rarer causes of intrahepatic cholestasis.
     To confirm the diagnosis of intrahepatic cholestasis, liver biopsy may be required along with above mentioned investigation.[2]

CASE SCENARIO 2: CHOLESTASIS

A 39-year-old lady, with no comorbidity, presented with pain in right upper quadrant of the abdomen since yesterday, which started 30 minutes after taking meals and is continuous. Also, she had an episode of fever with chills, which did not subside with antipyretic. On further enquiry, she mentioned that she had similar kind of pain episodes twice in the past, one 4 months back and the last one was about 1 month back. On examination, she is febrile, dehydrated, and in agonizing pain. Her pulse is 112 beats/min with blood pressure (BP) of 108/64 mm Hg. She looks icteric and severe tenderness is seen in the right hypochondriac region.

1. **How would you approach this case?**

   She was immediately started on intravenous (IV) fluids and routine blood biochemistry was sent, which includes hemogram, liver profile, and renal profile along with two sets of blood culture.

   As mentioned in **Table 2**, from the history, it looks like she had extrahepatic cholestasis (presence of abdominal pain and fever).

   Ultrasonography (USG) of the abdomen to be done, which showed multiple gall bladder stones with two small calculi in distal common bile duct (CBD) with upstream CBD dilatation and intrahepatic biliary radicle dilatation.

   A broad-spectrum antibiotic to be started and MRCP to be done for biliary anatomy identification. An endoscopic retrograde cholangiopancreatography (ERCP) to be done with ductal clearance and patient to be posted for laparoscopic cholecystectomy.

   So, what are the causes of extrahepatic cholestasis?[3]

TABLE 2: Causes of extrahepatic cholestasis.

Benign causes	Malignant causes
Choledocholithiasis	Cholangiocarcinoma
Benign stricture of common bile duct (CBD) (postoperative)	Periampullary carcinoma
Chronic pancreatitis causing CBD stricture	Gall bladder cancer
Biliary ascariasis	Lymph node metastasis at porta
Mirizzi syndrome	Cancer in the head of pancreas

REFERENCES

1. Lala V, Zubair M, Minter DA. Liver Function Tests. [Updated 2023 Jul 30]. In: StatPearls [Internet]. Treasure Island (FL): StatPearls Publishing; 2023 Jan. Available from: https://www.ncbi.nlm.nih.gov/books/NBK482489/.
2. Kumar R, Mehta G, Jalan R. Acute-on-chronic liver failure. Clin Med (Lond). 2020;20(5):501-4.
3. Jenniskens M, Langouche L, Van den Berghe G. Cholestatic Alterations in the Critically Ill: Some New Light on an Old Problem. Chest. 2018;153(3):733-43.

3.7: PANCREATITIS

CASE SCENARIO

A 50-year-old female comes to the emergency room (ER) with severe abdominal pain. It started immediately after food intake. She has a history of gallbladder stones.

1. **What laboratory findings will help us to diagnose pancreatitis?**
   Diagnostic criteria for acute pancreatitis
   At least two of the following are required:[1,2]
   1. Elevation of lipase more than three times the upper limit of normal (i.e., >500 U/L)
   2. Characteristic abdominal pain
   3. Imaging evidence of pancreatitis on computed tomography (CT), magnetic resonance imaging (MRI), or ultrasound

   Lipase:
   - Sensitivity and specificity are ~90% for acute pancreatitis.
   - Elevations of lipase due to diseases other than pancreatitis tend to be under three times the upper limit of normal.
     - Very high lipase values are more *specific* for a diagnosis of pancreatitis.
     - Higher lipase values *do not* correlate with worse prognostic outcome.
   - Lipase has replaced amylase for the diagnosis of pancreatitis.

   Laboratory findings to evaluate the cause of pancreatitis:
   - *Calcium:* Hypercalcemia is a rare cause of pancreatitis.
   - *Triglyceride level:* >1,000 mg/dL suggests hypertriglyceridemic pancreatitis.
   - *Liver function tests:* Significantly elevated bilirubin and alkaline phosphatase suggest obstruction, raising a possible concern of simultaneous ascending cholangitis.
   - C-reactive protein (CRP).

REFERENCES

1. Wyncoll DLA. Severe acute pancreatitis. Oh's Intensive Care Manual. pp. 495.
2. Leppäniemi A, Tolonen M, Tarasconi A, Segovia-Lohse H, Gamberini E, Kirkpatrick AW, et al. 2019. WSES guidelines for the management of severe acute pancreatitis. World J Emerg Surg. 2019;14:27.

3.8: ACUTE CORONARY SYNDROME

CASE SCENARIO

A 46-year-old gentleman presented to the emergency room (ER) with chest pain.

1. **What laboratory evaluation should be done in this patient?**
   Cardiac troponin is currently the first-line test for evaluating patients with suspected acute myocardial infarction (AMI). Troponin T and troponin I levels in the blood rise as early as 4 hours from the onset of AMI symptoms, peaks in 24–48 hours, and remain elevated for multiple days, thereby making them useful for detecting initial ischemic events but not reliable to detect reinfarction. High-sensitivity troponin assay (hs-TnT), a test developed to detect troponin at much lower concentrations than what the conventional troponin tests can detect, allows for more rapid diagnosis in patients admitted to the hospital, suspected to have AMI. Researchers also noted that this test had 100% sensitivity and negative predictive value in diagnosing AMI, but the specificity was limited.

   The investigations of importance in acute coronary syndrome are creatine phosphokinase (CPK) MB, troponin T, and troponin I. Creatine kinase-MB (CK-MB) concentration gradually rises in blood in 4–6 hours after onset of chest pain, peaks by around 24 hours, and returns rapidly to baseline in 48 hours.

   Troponin elevation >99th percentile is used as the cutoff value for the diagnosis of AMI. Troponin concentration begins to rise 4–6 hours after onset of symptoms, peaks by about 18–24 hours, and remains in the detectable levels for 72–96 hours.

   Troponin is more specific to the cardiac muscle when compared to CK-MB, and current assays for troponin are more sensitive and specific than the assays for CK-MB measurement. Given the expression of CK-MB in skeletal muscle and the presence of evidence proving the failure of CK-MB relative index and several other non-AMI causes of CK-MB elevation, troponin has been proven as the biomarker of choice for the detection of myocardial damage of any etiology.

   Troponin remains in circulation for a longer duration when compared to CK-MB. In conditions where reinfarction is suspected, CK-MB may be useful to classify a new event due to its shorter duration of elevation at detectable levels in plasma.[1-3]

REFERENCES

1. Bhatt DL, Lopes RD, Harrington RA. Diagnosis and Treatment of Acute Coronary Syndromes: A Review. JAMA. 2022;327(7):662-75.
2. Shirodaria C, Dawkins S. Acute Coronary Syndromes. In: Davey P, Sprigings D (Eds). Diagnosis and Treatment in Internal Medicine (Oxford, 2018; online edn, Oxford Academic, 1 Aug. 2018), https://doi.org/10.1093/med/9780199568741.003.0090.
3. Wilcox HM, Vickery AW, Emery JD. Cardiac troponin testing for diagnosis of acute coronary syndromes in primary care. Med J Aust. 2015;203(8):336.

CHAPTER 4

Endocrinological Abnormalities

Gurudas Sadanand Pundpal, Rahul Anil Pandit

CASE SCENARIO 1: ADRENAL INSUFFICIENCY

A 23-year-old female admitted with 4 months history of persistent vomiting, initially thought because of gastritis, 6–8 episodes a day, and weight loss. She was lethargic and drowsy. In the emergency room (ER), the patient's blood pressure was 80 systolic and pulse rate was 114 beats/min. The patient was looking dehydrated with cold extremities. Fluid resuscitation with normal saline was started and she was shifted to critical care unit. Her hemoglobin was 12 g/dL, white blood cell (WBC) count 12,500/L, sodium 128 mEq/L, potassium 4.9 mEq/L, and C-reactive protein (CRP) 12. Arterial blood gas (ABG) analysis shows pH 7.42, partial pressure of carbon dioxide (PCO_2) 38, bicarbonate (HCO_3) 23, partial pressure of oxygen (PaO_2) 88, and lactate 2.4 with normal liver and renal function tests. Serum random cortisol level was requested in view of persistent hypotension despite adequate fluid resuscitation, which came back 9 µg/dL.

1. **What is the diagnosis?**
   Adrenal insufficiency—primary (Addison disease) or secondary adrenal insufficiency (pituitary issues).

2. **What is the clinical presentation of patient with adrenal insufficiency?**
   Most striking presentation of all the patients presenting to intensive care unit is adrenal crisis with shock refractory to fluid resuscitation and vasopressors and rapid improvement only following use of steroids. Secondary adrenal insufficiency has a similar presentation as that of primary adrenal insufficiency, except hyperpigmentation and absence of mineralocorticoid deficiency features, such as hyperkalemia.[1]

3. **What are the laboratory investigations that help us to diagnose adrenal insufficiency?**
   The laboratory findings include hyponatremia, hyperkalemia, and hypoglycemia. Hyponatremia is due to cortisol and aldosterone deficiency. Aldosterone deficiency causes sodium wasting, and cortisol deficiency results in increased antidiuretic hormone. This causes increased water absorption. Hypovolemia also triggers antidiuretic hormone (ADH) secretion. Hyperkalemia is secondary to low aldosterone levels, which causes natriuresis and potassium retention. Hyperkalemia does not occur in secondary disease; this helps to distinguish from primary adrenal insufficiency. Hypoglycemia is multifactorial, including decreased oral intake and lack of glucocorticoids, which are essential for gluconeogenesis. Hypoglycemia is multifactorial, including decreased oral

intake and lack of glucocorticoids, which are essential for gluconeogenesis. Hypercalcemia may be present, which reflects extracellular fluid loss.
- *Cortisol level:*
  - >18 µg/dL: Normal
  - <3 µg/dL: Adrenal insufficiency
  - 3–19 µg/dL: Equivocal and further evaluation is suggested.
- *Adrenocorticotropic hormone (ACTH) level and corticotropin stimulation test:*
  - Primary adrenal insufficiency: Elevated ACTH
  - Central adrenal insufficiency: Abnormally normal or low ACTH

  With ACTH stimulation:
  - *Normal response:* Adequate response (peak cortisol level >18 µg/dL)
  - *Adrenal insufficiency:* Less or no response

4. **How to manage a patient with adrenal insufficiency?**
Addison crisis is a severe endocrine emergency; immediate recognition and treatment are required. Beware that if not recognized and treated, the adrenal crisis can be fatal.
- Fluid resuscitation to restore the intravascular volume with intravenous (IV) normal saline.
- Dextrose to correct hypoglycemia
- Correction of the hormone deficiency, both glucocorticoid and mineralocorticoid

The immediate hormonal treatment is the administration of hydrocortisone. Hypoglycemia should be treated promptly.

Maintenance Phase
Life-long treatment with hormonal replacement is required. Maintenance therapy aims to provide a replacement to maintain a physiologic glucocorticoid and mineralocorticoid level. The usual doses are as follows:
- *Glucocorticoid:* Hydrocortisone 5–25 mg/day (can be divided into two or three doses) and prednisone 3–5 mg/day[2,3]
- *Mineralocorticoid:* Fludrocortisone 0.05–0.2 mg daily[2]

Treatment Considerations
In patients with Addison's disease, glucocorticoid secretion does not increase during stress. Therefore, in the presence of fever, infection, or other illnesses, the hydrocortisone dose should be increased to compensate for a possible stress response.[4]

CASE SCENARIO 2: CONN'S SYNDROME

A 37-year-old female, a known case of systemic hypertension, came to the ER with complaints of palpitation, headache, and shortness of breath since a week. In the ER, the patient was conscious and alert. Her pulse rate was 110 beats/min and blood pressure 180/110 mm Hg. Her systemic examination of respiratory, cardiovascular, and nervous system was unremarkable. Electrocardiography (ECG) was suggestive of left ventricular strain pattern. Her serum sodium was 136 mEq/L, potassium 2.9 mEq/L, and the rest of renal and liver functions were within normal range. The patient had uncontrolled hypertension despite of starting on three different antihypertensive medications—amlodipine, metoprolol, and telmisartan. She was on oral potassium supplement in view of low potassium levels. In view of drug-resistant hypertension and persistent hypokalemia, plasma aldosterone and renin activity were measured. Plasma aldosterone concentration (PAC) was 90 ng/dL and plasma renin activity (PRA) was 0.20 ng/mL/h with PAC/PRA ratio was 450. The elevated PAC/PAR ratio is suggestive of hyperaldosteronism, a contrast-enhanced computed tomography (CT) scan and magnetic resonance imaging (MRI) scan of abdomen done, suggestive of unilateral adenoma. Tablet spironolactone was started subsequently, which resulted into control of blood pressure and correction of serum potassium level.

1. **What is the diagnosis?**
   Conn's syndrome,

2. **What is Conn's syndrome?**
   Primary hyperaldosteronism (Conn's syndrome) is an endocrine disorder characterized by excessive aldosterone production from adrenal gland, resulting into reduced renin activity and uncontrolled hypertension.[5]

3. **What is the pathophysiology of Conn's syndrome?**
   Hyperaldosteronism results in hypokalemia, plasma volume expansion, hypertension, metabolic alkalosis, and reduced renin levels.

4. **How to diagnose Conn's syndrome?**
   - Hypokalemia in a hypertensive patient is the most common clue for primary hyperaldosteronism. However, normal serum potassium may be present in up to 38% of patients, especially in patients with adrenal hyperplasia or familial aldosteronism.
   - *ABG:* Hypokalemia, hypernatremia, and metabolic alkalosis are due to the actions of aldosterone on the distal convoluted tubule.
   - Urinary potassium excretion is elevated (>30 mmol/day).
   - *Aldosterone:renin ratio:* A ratio of 40 or more (20–40 ng/dL/h) or >135 (68–135 pmol/mU) has a sensitivity of 73–93% and a specificity of 71–84%, indicating the need for further confirmatory studies with salt loading (failure to lower plasma aldosterone level <10 ng/dL), fludrocortisone suppression test, or captopril suppression test. If screening test is suggestive of primary hyperaldosteronism, then confirmatory diagnostic tests are performed, including 24-hour urinary aldosterone excretion test, ambulatory salt-loading test, or fludrocortisone suppression test.

5. **How to treat Conn's syndrome?**
   The primary goals of treatment of primary aldosteronism are normalization of blood pressure, potassium level, and aldosterone activity.[6,7]

   Surgical treatment: Unilateral adrenalectomy in patients with a unilateral adenoma (Conn's syndrome) cures hypertension.

Endocrinological Abnormalities

CASE SCENARIO 3: HYPEROSMOLAR HYPERGLYCEMIC STATE

A 56-year-old female, a known case of type II diabetes mellitus, presented with complaints of fever and burning sensation while passing urine. The patient had pain in abdomen, multiple episodes of vomiting, and breathing difficulty. The patient was a diagnosed case of type II diabetes mellitus and had history of poor glycemic control. On clinical examination, the patient was febrile. She was clinically dehydrated with a dry tongue and reduced skin turgor. There was tachycardia of 130 beats/min with blood pressure of 90/60 mm Hg and respiratory rate was 24 cycles/min. The chest was clear on auscultation.

1. **What is the diagnosis?**
   Hyperosmolar hyperglycemic state (HHS).

2. **What are the characteristic features of HHS?**
   - Hypovolemia—severely dehydrated and unwell
   - Marked hyperglycemia (>30 mmol/L) without significant ketonuria (<3 mmol/L) or acidosis (pH > 7.3 and bicarbonate > 15 mmol/L)
   - Osmolality is usually 320 mOsm/kg or more.

		Reference values
pH	7.35	7.35–7.45
PaO_2 (mm Hg)	103	83–108
$PaCO_2$ (mm Hg)	38	32–48
HCO_3^- (mmol/L)	23	22–28
Glucose (mg/dL)	786	65–95
Lactate (mmol/L)	2.2	0.4–0.8
Sodium (mmol/L)	150	136–145
Potassium (mmol/L)	4.5	3.4–4.5
Chloride (mmol/L)	106	98–107
Creatinine (mg/dL)	2.5	0.45–1.09

3. **What are the most common precipitants of HHS?**
   Infection, inadequate or missed insulin doses, pancreatitis, myocardial infarction, cerebrovascular accident, and drugs (e.g., corticosteroids, thiazides, and sympathomimetics) are the most common precipitants of HHS.

4. **Why are ketone bodies absent in HHS?**
   Relative insulin deficiency results in hyperglycemia and subsequent osmotic diuresis. However, insulin levels are adequate to prevent lipolysis and hepatic ketogenesis.[8]

5. **What are the signs of severe HHS?**
   - Osmolality >350 mOsmol/kg
   - Sodium above 160 mmol/L
   - Venous/arterial pH below 7.1

- Hypokalemia (<3.5 mmol/L) or hyperkalemia (>6 mmol/L) on admission
- Glasgow Coma Scale (GCS) < 12
- Oxygen saturation below 92% on air (assuming normal baseline respiratory function)
- Systolic blood pressure below 90 mm Hg
- Pulse over 100 or below 60 beats/min
- Urine output <0.5 mL/kg/h
- Serum creatinine above 200 µmol/L
- Hypothermia
- Macrovascular event, such as myocardial infarction or stroke.

6. **What are the principles of management of HHS?**

   The key principles of management of HHS are:
   - Replace fluid and electrolyte losses
   - Slowly restore osmolality and glucose to normal levels
   - Prevent secondary complications.

7. **How to do fluid management?**
   - Expect a 200 mL/kg total water deficit.
   - *Commence fluid resuscitation:*
     - 15–20 mL/kg in the first hour
     - 4–14 mL/kg in the second hour (of 0.45% NaCl)
     - 4–14 mL/kg again in the third hour (use 0.9% NaCl if the sodium is low)
     - When glucose is under 15 mmol/L, start 5% dextrose 100–250 mL/h

   Fluid resuscitation will bring down sugar. Insulin therapy may not be required and may even be dangerous.

   In HHS, the serum glucose level will often fall with initial fluid resuscitation, and patients are normally highly insulin sensitive. Therefore, there is a risk of a precipitous initial fall in blood glucose and serum osmolality. Consequently, the presence of relative hypoinsulinemia should be identified by testing for significant ketonemia (blood 3-beta-hydroxybutyrate > 1 mmol/L). Only if this is present should insulin be started? For all other patients, insulin is only introduced when the rate of fall of glucose from fluid resuscitation has reached a plateau. Where insulin is started, the dose is reduced in HHS to 0.05 units/kg as a fixed rate insulin infusion. A maximum decrease in blood glucose of 5 mmol/L/h should be targeted.

8. **What is the target serum osmolarity?**

   Serum sodium will inevitably rise due to the movement of water back into the intracellular space. A sodium rise of 2.4 mmol/L occurs for each 5.5 mmol/L fall in glucose. A safe drop is 3–8 mOsm/kg/h. Excessively rapid correction places the patient at risk of neurological complications, such as central pontine myelinolysis and cerebral edema.

9. **How do you calculate serum osmolality?**

   Calculated osmolality = 2Na + glucose + urea

   Excessively rapid correction places the patient at risk of neurological complications, such as central pontine myelinolysis and cerebral edema.

10. What are the complications of HHS?

The complications are as:
- Thromboembolism
- Cerebral complications—confusion, decreased consciousness, seizures, cerebral edema, and central pontine myelinolysis.

CASE SCENARIO 4: DIABETIC KETOACIDOSIS

A 56-year-old female, a known case of type II diabetes mellitus, presented with complaints of fever and burning sensation while passing urine. The patient had pain in abdomen, multiple episodes of vomiting, and breathing difficulty. The patient was diagnosed with a case of type II diabetes mellitus and had a history of poor glycemic control. On clinical examination, the patient was febrile. She was clinically dehydrated with a dry tongue and reduced skin turgor. There was tachycardia of 130 beats/min with blood pressure of 90/60 mm Hg and respiratory rate was 24 breaths/min. The chest was clear on auscultation.

The ABG analysis is as follows:

		Reference values
pH	7.06	7.35–7.45
PaO$_2$ (mm Hg)	80	83–108
PaCO$_2$ (mm Hg)	22	32–48
HCO$_3^-$ (mmol/L)	9	22–28
Glucose (mg/dL)	450	65–95
Lactate (mmol/L)	1.2	0.4–0.8
Sodium (mmol/L)	128	136–145
Potassium (mmol/L)	3.2	3.4–4.5
Chloride (mmol/L)	96	98–107
Creatinine (mg/dL)	1.12	0.45–1.09

1. What is the diagnosis?

Diabetic ketoacidosis (DKA).

2. What are the key elements of pathophysiology?

The key elements of pathophysiology of DKA are:[9]
- *Insulin deficiency and hyperglycemia:* Insulin deficiency leads to increased secretion of glucagon, which accelerates hepatic glucose production. As a result of increased production and decreased metabolism, blood glucose level increases.
- *Ketosis and metabolic acidosis:* As glucose cannot be utilized as a source of energy, increased lipolysis provides free fatty acids as a source of energy. Glucagon converts free fatty acids into ketone bodies in the liver. Predominant ketone bodies are beta-hydroxybutyrate and acetoacetic acid. Increased production of ketone bodies leads to high anion gap metabolic acidosis.

- *Fluid and electrolyte abnormalities:* Hyperglycemia-induced osmotic diuresis leads to loss of water and electrolytes. Severe hyperglycemia results into fluid loss of about 6–8 liters in patients with DKA. Osmotic diuresis also causes marked depletion of electrolytes, such as sodium, potassium, chloride, magnesium, and phosphate. Although, there is depletion of fluid and electrolytes in DKA, serum electrolytes may be within normal range due to shift of water and electrolytes from intracellular to extracellular compartment as a result of increased serum osmolality due to hyperglycemic state and metabolic acidosis.[10]

3. **What is the clinical presentation of DKA?**
   There is severe dehydration, dry skin and tongue, loss of skin turgor, sunken eyeballs, and reduced urine output. Patients have tachycardia, deep and labored breathing, also called Kussmaul's breathing with fruity odor of acetone in the breath. Patients with DKA are often lethargic. If untreated at this stage, the patient may progress to coma and hypotension, leading to circulatory failure and death.

   Indications for critical care admission are as follows:
   - Blood ketones > 6 mmol/L
   - Bicarbonate level < 5 mmol/L
   - Venous/arterial pH < 7.0
   - Hypokalemia on admission (under 3.5 mmol/L)
   - GCS < 12
   - Oxygen saturation below 92% on air (assuming normal baseline respiratory function)
   - Systolic blood pressure below 90 mm Hg
   - Pulse over 100 or below 60 beats/min
   - Anion gap above 16 [Anion gap = (Na + K) − (Cl + HCO_3)].

4. **How do you diagnose DKA?**
   Laboratory investigation findings in DKA are as follows:
   - *Blood glucose level:* Blood glucose concentration in DKA is typically in the range of 400–600 mg/dL. Some cases of DKA present with blood sugar level < 300 mg/dL, also called euglycemic DKA.
   - *Renal function tests:* Blood urea nitrogen (BUN) and creatinine are typically elevated in patients with DKA.
   - *Serum electrolytes:*
     - *Sodium:* Serum sodium level is variable ranging from 120 to 160 mEq/L in patients with DKA. Elevated sodium level reflects the degree of free water loss and dehydration. Shift of free water from intracellular to extracellular compartment because of osmotic gradient created by hyperglycemia result in abnormally low serum sodium concentration. There is a fall in measured sodium concentration by 1.6 mEq/L with each 100 mg/dL increase in blood sugar above 100 mg/dL. Corrected sodium levels should be calculated in all patients with DKA.
     - *Potassium:* At presentation, serum potassium levels are usually elevated in patients with DKA due to dehydration and shift of potassium from intracellular to extracellular compartment due to severe metabolic acidosis. Serum potassium

levels should be monitored closely during treatment of DKA because after initiation of insulin therapy, there is intracellular shift of potassium, leading to precipitous fall in serum potassium concentration. Prompt correction of potassium level is necessary during treatment, otherwise cardiac arrhythmias may be precipitated due to hypokalemia.
- *Magnesium:* Similar to potassium, magnesium concentration is usually elevated in initial presentation, but it falls with initiation of treatment.
- *Phosphate:* During the course of correction, phosphate levels also should be monitored and corrected as phosphate is an important component of adenosine triphosphate (ATP) production.
- *Arterial blood gas and ketone bodies:* Arterial blood pH is always <7.3 in patients with DKA and usually <7.0 in cases of severe DKA. DKA is typically present with high anion gap metabolic acidosis. Rarely metabolic alkalosis may accompany anion gap acidosis due to severe vomiting in patients with DKA. Serum ketone bodies are always present in DKA. Commonly done test to measure ketone bodies is nitroprusside test, which measures only acetoacetate and acetone and does not measure beta-hydroxybutyrate.
- *Complete blood count:* Hemoglobin and hematocrit levels are usually elevated in initial stages of DKA due to plasma volume contraction. WBC count is always elevated even in the absence of infection.
- *Urine analysis:* Urine ketone should be checked as part of initial diagnosis algorithm. Urinary ketones should not be used to guide treatment as they will remain positive even after the DKA has resolved.

5. **How do you manage a patient with DKA?**

   The principles of management of DKA are as follows:
   - Fluid resuscitation
   - Replacement of electrolytes
   - Insulin therapy
   - Treatment of precipitation factors

   Patients with DKA should be admitted to the intensive care unit. Treatment of DKA is directed toward replacement of fluid, electrolytes, and insulin in that order.
   - *Fluid resuscitation:* Newer studies advocate the use of the balanced salt solution to maintain the electrolyte hemostasis. Further, fluid replacement rate should be determined by patient's clinical response and urine output. About 75% of fluid deficit should be corrected in the first 24 hours. After initial fluid resuscitation, the replacement fluid may be changed to 1–2 liters of 0.45% saline in patients with hypernatremia. Once plasma glucose level falls to 180–200 mg/dL, 0.9% saline should be replaced by 5% or 10% dextrose for fluid replacement to prevent hypoglycemia. IV insulin therapy needs to be continued as ketogenesis continues despite a fall in plasma glucose level.
   - *Replacement of electrolytes:*
     - *Potassium:* Although the initial serum potassium level is normal, there is significant total body potassium deficit in DKA. Once fluid and insulin replacement have started, serum potassium levels fall and frequently become subnormal during

treatment of DKA. Prompt replacement of potassium with IV potassium chloride is necessary. Severe hypokalemia can precipitate life-threatening cardiac arrhythmia. Serum potassium levels and ECG should be monitored periodically during treatment. Rate of potassium replacement is adjusted according to serum potassium levels.
- *Phosphate:* Serum phosphate concentration falls during treatment of DKA. Although, serum phosphate falls below the normal level, phosphate replacement is rarely needed in patients with severe hypophosphatemia (<1.0 mg/dL). Potassium phosphate is used for phosphate replacement whenever necessary. Severe hypophosphatemia can lead to muscle weakness, respiratory failure due to involvement of respiratory muscles, rhabdomyolysis, and depressed cardiac contractility and neurological disturbances.
- *Bicarbonate:* Even if patients with DKA present with metabolic acidosis, bicarbonate therapy is not needed for correction of acidosis. In fact, bicarbonate treatment may have deleterious effects, such as worsening hypokalemia, late metabolic alkalosis, and cerebral edema, especially in children.

- *Insulin therapy:* Insulin should be provided via a weight-based fixed-rate intravenous insulin infusion (FRIII). Insulin at 0.1 units/kg should be started as soon as fluid resuscitation is commenced.

  Blood glucose levels should be monitored every 1–2 hours initially. Insulin infusion is titrated to achieve fall in blood glucose level at a rate of 75–100 mg/dL. Target blood sugar level in the first 24 hours is between 150 and 200 mg/dL. Both hypoglycemia and development of hyperglycemia should be avoided. Even if blood sugar falls below 200 mg/dL, insulin infusion should be continued as ketogenesis may continue despite normalization of blood sugar level. Hypoglycemia is prevented by replacing 0.9% saline with 5% or 10% dextrose solution for fluid replacement.

  Arterial blood gas analysis for resolution of acidosis and normalization of anion gap guides about clearance of ketosis. Once the anion gap is normalized, the patient is conscious, alert, clinically stable, and is able to eat and drink. Insulin treatment with subcutaneous insulin is started. Insulin infusion should be continued till onset of action of subcutaneous insulin.

- *Treatment of precipitation factors:* Identification of precipitating factor and appropriate treatment of same is very important. Active search for presence of infection should be done in each case of DKA.

6. **What are the complications associated with DKA?**

   Complications associated with DKA are:
   - *Hypoglycemia:* To prevent hypoglycemia, it is advisable to keep blood glucose level close to 200 mg/dL in the first 24 hours. If blood glucose level falls below 200 mg/dL, replacement fluid is changed to 5% dextrose instead of normal saline.
   - Cerebral edema
   - Thrombotic complications
   - Renal failure.

CASE SCENARIO 5: HYPOGLYCEMIA

A 64-year-old male patient, a known case of type II diabetes mellitus, on oral hypoglycemic treatment, was brought by relatives with history of sudden-onset altered sensorium. Relatives denied history of headache, vomiting, head injury, or witnessed seizure. In the ER, the patient was drowsy, difficult to arouse. There was no neck stiffness and no focal neuro deficit. He was not obeying commands and was afebrile. His pulse rate was 112 beats/min with sinus tachycardia, blood pressure 90/50 mm Hg, and respiratory rate 22 breaths/min. His laboratory investigations were as follows: Hemoglobin 10 g/dL and WBC 12×10^9/L. Liver function test was essentially normal, creatinine was 2.3 mg/dL, and BUN 34 mg/dL. Blood sugar was 36 mg/dL. Immediately 50 mL of 50% dextrose was infused to patient. The patient became conscious and alert post dextrose infusion. On detailed history taking, history of fever and burning micturition was present since last 4 days. Relatives also gave history of reduced oral intake and decreases urine output since last 2 days.

		Reference values
pH	7.39	7.35–7.45
PaO$_2$ (mm Hg)	80	83–108
PaCO$_2$ (mm Hg)	22	32–48
HCO$_3^-$ (mmol/L)	24	22–28
Glucose (mg/dL)	36	65–95
Lactate (mmol/L)	1.2	0.4–0.8
Sodium (mmol/L)	138	136–145
Potassium (mmol/L)	3.9	3.4–4.5
Chloride (mmol/L)	104	98–107
Creatinine (mg/dL)	2.3	0.45–1.09

1. **What is hypoglycemia?**
   Hypoglycemia is not defined by any specific blood sugar level. The Whipple's triad of hypoglycemia consists of:
   - Documentation of low blood glucose level
   - Presence of symptoms consistent with hypoglycemia
   - Resolution of hypoglycemic symptoms post glucose administration.

2. **What are the causes for development of hypoglycemia?**
   Hormonal imbalance principally involving insulin is most common cause of hypoglycemia.[11]
   - Insulin overdose (iatrogenic)
   - Insulin secreting tumors—insulinoma and insulin-secreting nonislet tumor
   - Hypoglycemia with use of oral hypoglycemic agents—some of the sulfonylureas have half-life >24 hours. Prolongation of duration of action due to hepatic or renal dysfunction can result in prolonged hypoglycemia.

3. **Which drugs other than insulin can cause hypoglycemia?**
   - Ethanol causes hypoglycemia by suppressing hepatic gluconeogenesis.
   - Beta-blocker agents—noncardioselective agents such as propranolol and nadolol may precipitate hypoglycemia.
   - Antiarrhythmic agents—quinidine is known to cause hypoglycemia in susceptible individuals.
   - Other agents rarely causing hypoglycemia include salicylates, angiotensin-converting enzyme (ACE) inhibitors, and antibiotics such as pentamidine and gatifloxacin.

4. **How to manage a patient with hypoglycemia?**
   All comatose patients' blood sugar should be checked with finger-prick test and IV glucose should be administered promptly, if hypoglycemia is present. 50 mL of 50% dextrose solution is administered over the period of 2–5 minutes as an initial bolus in comatose patients. Rapid improvement in sensorium following glucose administration confirms hypoglycemia as a cause for altered sensorium. Oral glucose is preferred in alert and cooperative patients. After initial bolus dose of glucose, an infusion of 5% or 10% dextrose should be started to maintain blood glucose level around 100 mg/dL. If hypoglycemia is due to overdose of long-acting insulin, initial bolus dose of 50% dextrose should be followed by continuous infusion of 5–10% dextrose.[12,13]

5. **What blood investigations will you do in a patient with hypoglycemia?**
   In all patients with symptomatic hypoglycemia, blood glucose measurement should be done in clinical laboratory. Other laboratory tests to determine the cause of hypoglycemia include renal and liver function tests. In all the patients with hypoglycemic coma serum and plasma, samples are collected for measurement of C-peptide and proinsulin levels, if clinically indicated.

6. **How do you manage sulfonylurea-induced hypoglycemia?**
   If sulfonylureas are a cause for development of hypoglycemia, patient should be hospitalized as these agents have long duration of action. Activated charcoal may prevent absorption of the drug from the stomach, while alkalinization of urine may enhance excretion of the drug. Sulfonylurea-induced hypoglycemia typically takes 2–3 days to resolve.

7. **How is persistent hypoglycemia treated?**
   - Continuous IV dextrose supplementation
   - Glucocorticoids
   - Octreotide
   - Diazoxide.

REFERENCES

1. Cooper MS, Stewart PM. Corticosteroid insufficiency in acutely ill patients. N Engl J Med. 2003;348:727-34.
2. Annane D, Sebille V, Charpentier C, Bollaert P-E, François B, Korach J-M, et al. Effect of treatment with low dose of hydrocortisone and fludrocortisone on mortality in patients with septic shock. JAMA. 2002;288:862-71.

3. Sprung CL, Annane D, Keh D, Moreno R, Singer M, Freivogel K, et al. Hydrocortisone therapy for patients with septic shock. N Engl J Med. 2008;358:111-24.
4. Munir S, Rodriguez BSQ, Waseem M. Addison Disease. In: StatPearls [Internet]. Treasure Island (FL): StatPearls Publishing; 2022.
5. Byrd JB, Turcu AF, Auchus RJ. Primary Aldosteronism Practical Approach to Diagnosis and management. Circulation. 2018;138:823-35.
6. Chao C-T, Wu V-C, Kuo C-C, Lin Y-H, Chang C-C, Chueh SJ, et al. Diagnosis and management of primary aldosteronism: An updated review. Ann Med. 2013;45(4):375-83.
7. Parmar MS, Singh S. Conn Syndrome. In: StatPearls [Internet]. Treasure Island (FL): StatPearls Publishing; 2022.
8. French EK, Donihi AC, Korytkowski MT. Diabetic ketoacidosis and hyperosmolar hyperglycemic syndrome: Review of acute decompensated diabetes in adult patients. BMJ. 2019;365:l1114.
9. Perilli G, Saraceni C, Daniels MN, Ahmad A. Diabetic Ketoacidosis: A Review and Update. Curr Emerg Hosp Med Rep. 2013;1:10-7.
10. Kamel KS, Halperin ML. Acid–Base problems in diabetic ketoacidosis. N Engl J Med. 2015;372:546-54.
11. Mordes JP, Thompson MJ, Harlan DH, Malkani S. Hypoglycemia. Irwin and Rippe's Intensive Care Medicine, 7th edition. Philadelphia: Wolters Kluwer Health/Lippincott Williams & Wilkins; 2012. pp. 1168-82.
12. Tourkmani AM, Alharbi TJ, Rsheed AMB, AlRasheed AN, AlBattal SM, Abdelhay O, et al. Hypoglycemia in type 2 Diabetes Mellitus patients: A review article. Diabetes Metab Syndr. 2018;12(5):791-4.
13. American Diabetes Association. Glycemic Targets: Standards of Medical Care in Diabetes—2020. Diabetes Care. 2020;43(Suppl 1):S66-76.

CHAPTER 5

Toxicology

PragnaSree R, Charudatt Vaity

INTRODUCTION

Toxicological analysis using blood or urine is used to confirm the diagnosis of poisoning when this is in doubt or for medicolegal purposes. Any toxicology screen should be tailored to that patient's circumstances and the poisons commonly encountered in that country. For patients, who present a complex clinical picture or who are unconscious, a 50 mL sample of urine and a 10 mL sample of heparinized blood should be collected on admission and stored at 4°C. This can be analyzed later if it is felt that the result will influence your management or is needed for medicolegal purposes. Urine is useful for screening, especially for drugs of abuse. Urine samples usually provide qualitative results, e.g., detect the presence of amphetamines or benzodiazepines. Quantitative measurements in urine are of little use because some compounds, such as benzodiazepines, are extensively metabolized prior to excretion in urine.

CASE SCENARIO 1: PYROGLUTAMIC ACIDOSIS

You are asked to review a 75-year-old female admitted for management of septic arthritis, affecting a prosthetic left hip joint inserted 2 years ago. She underwent debridement of the joint and antibiotic wash. Intraoperative specimens grew methicillin-sensitive *Staphylococcus aureus* and were started on intravenous (IV) flucloxacillin. She is on regular paracetamol for pain. Her past medical history was unremarkable and is not on any regular prescription medications. On day 10, she has continued to deteriorate and now has bilateral patchy infiltrates on her chest X-ray. She is on noninvasive ventilation (NIV) with 50% FiO_2.

Her vital signs were as follows: Heart rate (HR) 118 beats/min, blood pressure (BP) 107/58 mm Hg, respiratory rate (RR) 35 breaths/min, oxygen saturation (SpO_2) 100% on fraction of inspired oxygen (FiO_2) 0.6, and Glasgow Coma Scale (GCS) 12. Temperature 36.8°C. Rest of the examination was unremarkable. Her arterial blood gas (ABG) analysis is as follows:

		Reference values
pH	7.154	7.35–7.45
PaO_2 (mm Hg)	108	83–108
$PaCO_2$ (mm Hg)	27	32–48
HCO_3^- (mmol/L)	9	22–28
Glucose (mg/dL)	165	65–95
Lactate (mmol/L)	1.0	0.4–0.8

Contd...

Contd...

		Reference values
Sodium (mmol/L)	142	136–145
Potassium (mmol/L)	3.4	3.4–4.5
Chloride (mmol/L)	105	98–107
Creatinine (mg/dL)	1.6	0.45–1.09
Lactate (mmol/L)	1.2	0.45–1.09

1. **Describe the acid–base disturbance in the above ABG and calculate the anion gap.**
   Severe acidemia (pH 7.15) resulting from a high anion gap metabolic acidosis (HAGMA) with incomplete respiratory compensation.[1]
   Anion gap = [Na] − ([HCO$_3$] + [Cl]); normal anion gap is 2–10 mEq/L
   In this case, the anion gap is high: 142 − (8 + 104) = 30 mEq/L.

2. **List the likely causes of the primary acid–base disturbance. How would you confirm it?**
   Remember the common causes of HAGMA: CAT-MUDPILES (mnemonic)
   Given that the lactate and ketones are normal the most likely cause is *pyroglutamic acidemia* (aka 5-oxoprolinemia). This can be confirmed by performing a metabolic screen for urinary organic acids. Blood levels may be required if the patient is anuric. An elevated level of pyroglutamic acid confirms the diagnosis.[2]

3. **What is the underlying mechanism of pyroglutamic acidosis?**
   Pyroglutamic acidosis is a rare cause of HAGMA.[3] Pyroglutamic acid is also known as 5-oxoprolinemia. Its mechanism is as:
   - Produced from γ-glutamyl cysteine by the enzyme γ-glutamyl cyclotransferase
   - Catabolized by 5-oxoprolinase
   - When glutathione levels are low, the activity of γ-glutamyl cyclotransferase is increased, resulting in pyroglutamic acid accumulation in glutathione-depleted states.

4. **List the possible causes and risk factors of pyroglutamic acidosis.**
   - *Drugs:*
     - Paracetamol—depletion of glutathione by its metabolite N-acetyl-*p*-benzoquinone imine (NAPQI)
     - Flucloxacillin—inhibition of 5-oxoprolinase
     - Vigabatrin
   - *Severe sepsis:* Depletion of hepatic glutathione pools due to oxidative stress from stimulated leukocytes, reperfusion of ischemic tissue, or endotoxemia
   - *Organ dysfunction*—hepatic and renal
   - *Other*—malnutrition, pregnancy, and elderly patients
   - *Congenital enzyme deficiencies,* e.g., glutathione synthetase deficiency (mental retardation, hemolytic anemia, and metabolic acidosis).

5. **How do you manage this patient?**
   - Stop exacerbating factors
   - Treat sepsis including early and appropriate antibiotics and source control
   - Supportive care and monitoring—intubation, ventilation, renal replacement therapy (RRT) as indicated
   - N-acetylcysteine (NAC) helps to replenish glutathione stores.

CASE SCENARIO 2: LITHIUM

A 56-year-old female was brought to the emergency room (ER) with complaints of altered mental status and irrelevant speech since 4 hours ago. She is a known case of bipolar disorder since 25 years well controlled on lithium 800 mg once daily; no other significant medical history noted. There is no history of similar episodes in the past.

Arterial blood gas on admission was as follows—pH 7.35, partial pressure of oxygen (PO$_2$) 118 mm Hg, partial pressure of carbon dioxide (PCO$_2$) 42 mm Hg, HCO$_3^-$ 26 mmol/L, Na$^+$ 136 mmol/L, K$^+$ 5.6 mmol/L, chloride 118 mmol/L, creatinine 4.8 mg/dL, and lactate 1.2 mmol/L. Neuroimaging of the brain did not reveal any abnormality and lithium levels were 4.8 mEq/L.

1. **List the possible differential diagnosis.**
   - Manic/hypomanic relapse of bipolar disorder
   - Acute hyperactive delirium
   - Lithium toxicity[4]
   - Intoxication
   - Electrolyte disturbance
   - Cerebrovascular accident
   - Central nervous system (CNS) infection.

2. **Describe the pathophysiology of lithium toxicity.**
   - *Excessive intake:* Suicidal intent or accidental ingestion of excessive amounts of lithium tablets result in acute or acute-on-chronic overdose.
   - *Impaired excretion:* Sodium and volume depletion due to any conditions such as vomiting, diarrhea, febrile illness, renal insufficiency, excessive exercise, water restriction, excessive sweating, low sodium diet, and congestive heart failure may enhance lithium reabsorption in the kidneys. Chronic therapy with lithium can precipitate nephrogenic diabetes insipidus (NDI), resulting diminished urinary concentrating capacity of the kidneys.

3. **Discuss the pharmacokinetics of lithium.**
   - *Absorption:* Lithium is readily absorbed from the gastrointestinal (GI) tract with bioavailability close to 100% and peak plasma levels attained within 2-4 hours.
   - *Distribution:* It has small volume of distribution with no protein binding and exhibits slow entry into intracellular compartment (to exert the clinical effects). It is susceptible to accumulation in the liver, bone, muscle, or thyroid with brain and kidney showing the highest levels.
   - *Metabolism:* None

- *Excretion:* It is excreted 95% by kidneys and the rest is removed through sweat and feces. The renal clearance of lithium is usually 10–40 mL/min. The serum elimination half-life of lithium can vary from 12 to 27 hours. In chronic intoxication, the half-life can be prolonged up to 48 hours. Lithium freely crosses the placenta and is also excreted in breast milk. It is pregnancy class D and implicated in the increased risk of congenital cardiac defects, particularly the Ebstein anomaly.

4. **List the systemic effects of lithium toxicity.**
   - *Neurologic effects:* These include tremors, hyperreflexia, nystagmus, ataxia, and varying consciousness levels, ranging from mild confusion to delirium. Fine tremors are noted side effects of lithium therapy, while toxicity presents as coarse tremors. Syndrome of Irreversible Lithium-Effectuated Neurotoxicity (SILENT) defined as prolonged neurological complications of lithium toxicity, most commonly persistent cerebellar signs despite discontinuation of the medication and normalization of serum lithium levels.[5]
   - *Renal toxicity:* It includes impaired urinary concentrating ability, NDI (the most common cause of drug-induced NDI), sodium-losing nephritis, and nephrotic syndrome.
   - *Cardiovascular effects:* T-wave flattening is seen in most patients. Sinus node dysfunction is the most common reported conduction defect followed by QT prolongation, intraventricular conduction defects, and U waves.
   - *Gastrointestinal effects:* Nausea, vomiting, and abdominal discomfort are the GI effects. Symptoms typically occur within 1 hour of ingestion and are more common in the acute overdose setting.
   - *Endocrine effects:* Lithium administration leads to the inhibition of thyroid hormone synthesis and subsequent release, resulting in hypothyroidism.

5. **Discuss the classification of severity of lithium toxicity.**
   Lithium has a narrow therapeutic index.
   - *Therapeutic range of serum lithium levels:* 0.6–1.2 mEq/L
   - *Maintenance therapy:* 0.6–0.8 mEq/L
   - *Acute mania:* 1.0–1.2 mEq/L
   - Toxicity > 1.5 mEq/L

   Measurement of the serum levels should be carried out at least 6–12 hours after the last therapeutic dose to avoid misinterpretation of predistributional levels. The severity of lithium toxicity is often divided into the following three grades: mild, moderate, and severe.
   - *Mild symptoms:* Nausea, vomiting, lethargy, tremor, and fatigue (serum lithium concentration between 1.5 and 2.5 mEq/L)
   - *Moderate intoxication:* Confusion, agitation, delirium, tachycardia, and hypertonia (serum lithium concentration between 2.5 and 3.5 mEq/L)
   - *Severe intoxication:* Coma, seizures, hyperthermia, and hypotension (serum lithium concentration (>3.5 mEq/L).

6. **What are the expected changes on ABG in case of lithium toxicity?**
   Lithium toxicity per se is known to cause low to negative anion gap metabolic acidosis by contributing to unmeasured cations.

Other causes of a negative anion gap are as follows:
- Increase in unmeasured cations—lithium, polymyxin B, magnesium, and calcium
- Interference with the measurement of chloride, iodide, and bromide.

7. **Outline the treatment of lithium toxicity.**
   All patients with toxicity signs and symptoms, even those with normal serum lithium levels, should be admitted for monitoring in the hospital.
   - *Resuscitation:* Check airway, breathing, and circulation (ABC).
   - *Treat the underlying cause:* Infection, volume depletion, gastroenteritis, overdose, chronic kidney disease, drugs: NSAIDs, diuretics, cyclosporine, tetracyclines, decreased Na^+ intake, and anorexia.
   - Consider whole bowel irrigation for massive acute ingestion.
   - Activated charcoal does not bind—can be used in case of unknown coingestants.
   - Liberal fluid resuscitation with normal saline. Avoid hyponatremia as this will decrease lithium clearance.
   - Definitive management—hemodialysis (HD); peritoneal dialysis can be used if HD is not available.
   - Serial levels of lithium—every 6 hours in case of asymptomatic patients after acute ingestion. This should be continued until a declining trend has been established.
   - Patients should not be discharged until they are asymptomatic and have a serum lithium level less than 1.5 mEq/L.

CASE SCENARIO 3: TRICYCLIC ANTIDEPRESSANT TOXICITY

You are called to assess a 32-year-old female patient in the emergency department who was brought in a drowsy state, not obeying commands. She is tachycardic with a HR of 130 beats/min. The husband gives a history of ingestion of 50 tablets of amitriptyline of 25 mg strength.

Her ABG and electrocardiogram (ECG) obtained is as follows:

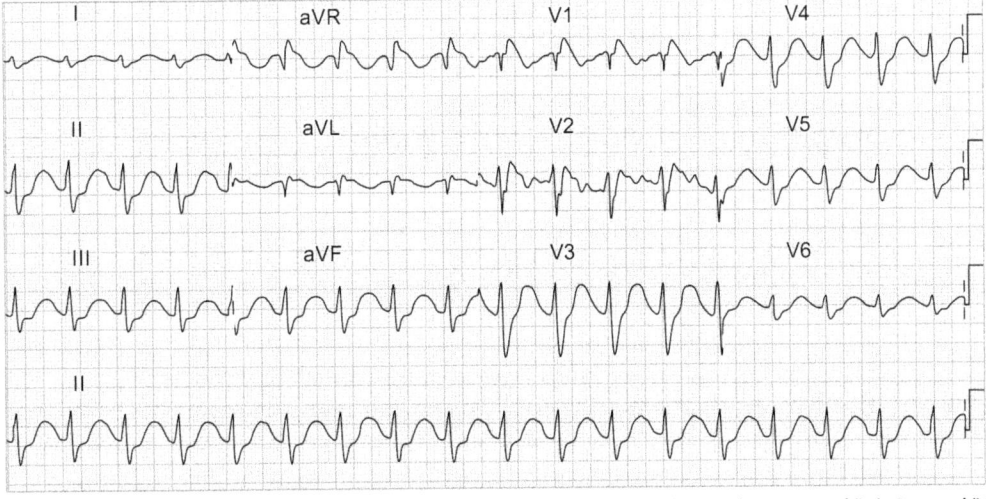

Vitals are as: pH 7.30, PO_2 123 mm Hg, PCO_2 32 mm Hg, HCO_3^- 17 mmol/L, and BE 8 mmol/L (±2 mmol/L)

1. **Discuss the ECG findings typical of tricyclic antidepressant (TCA) toxicity.**
   Most common ECG findings suggestive of TCA toxicity, indicative of sodium channel blockade, are:[6]
   - *QRS widening:*
     - >100 ms is associated with seizures
     - >160 ms is associated with cardiac dysrhythmias
   - Right axis deviation of the terminal QRS is defined by:
     - Terminal R wave >3 mm in aVR, or
     - R/S ratio >0.7 in aVR
   - Right bundle branch block (RBBB) pattern may be seen.
   - Tachycardia—due to anticholinergic effects of TCAs or as a reflex response to alpha1-blockade-mediated hypotension.
   - Bradycardia—generally a preterminal event

   In subtoxic doses or early presentation of toxicity, the ECG can be normal and needs to be closely monitored for QRS prolongation.

2. **Describe the mechanism of TCA toxicity.**
   Tricyclic antidepressants are weak bases (typically with pKa of ~8.5) that act as noradrenaline and serotonin reuptake inhibitors and gamma-aminobutyric acid A (GABA-A) receptor blockers.[7]

   Mechanism of toxicity includes:
   - Anticholinergic action
   - Inhibition of noradrenaline and serotonergic reuptake at nerve terminals
   - Direct alpha-adrenergic blockade
   - Membrane stabilizing effect on the myocardium by blockade of the cardiac and neurological fast sodium channels.

3. **Outline the systemic effects of TCA toxicity.**
   Systemic effects based on:
   - *Dose ingested:*[8]
     - >10 mg/kg is potentially life-threatening.
     - >30 mg/kg is expected to result in severe toxicity with pH-dependent cardiotoxicity and coma lasting for more than 24 hours.
     - Rapid deterioration within 1–2 hours of ingestion.
     - Delayed effects result from anticholinergic-mediated delayed gastric emptying or extended release amitriptyline.[9]
   - *Central nervous system:* Neurotoxicity precedes cardiotoxicity: sedation, delirium, seizures, and coma
   - *Cardiovascular system:*
     - Sinus tachycardia
     - Hypotension (alpha-blocking effects and myocardial depression)
     - Broad complex tachydysrhythmia (bradycardia occurs prearrest)
   - *Anticholinergic effects:* These are agitation, restlessness, delirium, mydriasis, dry, warm flushed skin, urinary retention, tachycardia, ileus, and myoclonic jerks.
   - Metabolic acidosis.

4. What is the specific antidote for TCA toxicity and its mechanism of action?
- Sodium bicarbonate is the antidote for TCA poisoning.
- Serum alkalization increases the proportion of nonionized form of the drug and reducing the amount of active form.
- The high sodium load increases the electrochemical gradient across cardiac cell membranes, potentially attenuating the TCA-induced blockade of sodium channels.

5. What is the end point of treatment with sodium bicarbonate?
Three end goals of sodium loading are:
1. Narrowing the QRS to <140 ms
2. Target Na^+ 155 mmol/L
3. pH aim of 7.5–7.55.

6. Outline the management of TCA toxicity.
- Assess and manage ABC
- Check ECG and ABG
- Consider gastric lavage/activated charcoal only if within 1 hour of potentially toxic dose and only after airway is secured.
- If intubated—consider hyperventilation to attain a pH of 7.5–7.55
- Seizures—IV benzodiazepines (e.g., midazolam 1–2 mg)
- Hypotension—crystalloid bolus (10–20 mL/kg), followed by vasopressor (e.g., noradrenaline infusion)
- Arrhythmias—avoid antiarrhythmic, correct hypoxia, hypotension, and acidosis
  - Class Ia and c antiarrhythmic drugs should be avoided—worsen sodium channel blockade, further slow conduction velocity, and depress contractility.
  - Class II agents (beta blockers)—precipitate hypotension and cardiac arrest.
- *Cardiac arrest/arrhythmia/hemodynamically unstable*—sodium bicarbonate 100 mEq/L (2 mEq/kg) bolus every few minutes while monitoring the effect on ECG until hemodynamically. Do not exceed dose of 6 mEq/kg.
- In case of *ongoing arrhythmia, QRS > 140 ms, or hypotension then* options include:
  - 3% saline can be given to achieve a sodium of 155 mmol/L if further bicarbonate cannot be given.
  - Lidocaine 1–1.5 mg/kg slow IV push, followed by 20–50 µg/kg/min infusion
  - Intralipid
  - Venoarterial extracorporeal membrane oxygenation (VA-ECMO).

CASE SCENARIO 4: PROPOFOL INFUSION SYNDROME

You are called to review a 30-year-old male patient with subarachnoid hemorrhage on mechanical ventilation with difficulty controlling BP. Patient is on infusion of fentanyl and midazolam. He is receiving multiple antihypertensives despite which the BP is still 190/110 mm Hg, and hence, propofol infusion was started. It has been 36 hours since the infusion and the nursing staff calls you with concern of green urine in the urometer.

1. **What are the causes of green-colored urine?**
   Oral or intravenous administration of substances containing phenol/thymol/chlorophyll can result in green urine. Drug culprits include cimetidine, amitriptyline, promethazine, propofol, triamterene, and methylene blue.

2. **What is propofol infusion syndrome and its pathophysiology?**
   - Propofol infusion syndrome (PRIS) is a potentially life-threatening condition seen in patients receiving high-dose propofol infusion (>4 mg/kg/h) for a prolonged duration (>48 hours).[10,11]
   - *Diagnostic criteria include:*
     - Sudden-onset bradycardia—resistant to treatment progressing to asystole.
       - ECG changes with Brugada-like pattern (coved ST changes—convex curved ST elevation in V1-V3) is characteristic in PRIS
     - Hypertriglyceridemia (lipemic serum)
     - Rhabdomyolysis
     - Acute renal failure
   - *Other clinical features include:*
     - Fatty liver and hepatomegaly
     - Coagulopathy
     - Raised plasma malonylcarnitine and C5 acylcarnitine
   - Unexplained new-onset metabolic acidosis and lactic acidosis are commonly noted.
   - PRIS is due to inhibition of coenzyme Q and cytochrome C by propofol, resulting in failure of electron transport chain and failure of ATP production. The fatty acid metabolism is impaired.
   - Propofol antagonizes β-adrenergic receptor and calcium channel binding hence depressing cardiac function.

3. **List the risk factors for developing PRIS.**
   Risk factors for developing PRIS include:
   - Young age children are more susceptible than adults due to lower glycogen stores and dependence on fat metabolism.
   - Traumatic brain injury
   - Sepsis
   - Catecholamine and/or glucocorticoid infusions
   - Low carbohydrate to high lipid intake
   - Inborn errors of fatty acid oxidation—medium chain acyl-CoA dehydrogenase (MCAD)
   - Propofol at dose >4 mg/kg/h for prolonged duration >48 hours (can occur at low doses as well)
   - Carnitine deficiency.

4. **Discuss the management of PRIS.**
   - High index of suspicion in at risk population
   - Monitor for early warning signs

- *Enhanced elimination:*
  - Discontinue propofol immediately
  - Hemodialysis and/or plasma exchange
- Specific antidote—carnitine (propofol infusion like syndrome is noted in response to lipid emulsion in the background of acquired carnitine deficiency)[12]
- *Supportive care:*
  - Adequate carbohydrate intake and minimizing lipid loads.
  - Consider pacing for bradycardia—shown limited success.
  - ECMO may be beneficial for cardiovascular support.

CASE SCENARIO 5: ETHYLENE GLYCOL POISONING

A 45-year-old male was brought to the ER in a stuporous and agitated state with history of consumption of 100 mL of radiator coolant 2 hours ago.

1. **What products typically contain ethylene glycol?**
   Ethylene glycol is a colorless, sweet tasting liquid. It is commonly found in radiator coolants, antifreeze solutions, brake fluids, and industrial solvents.[13]

2. **Discuss the mechanism of ethylene glycol toxicity.**
   Dose of 1-2 mL/kg of 95% concentrated ethylene glycol is considered a potentially life-threatening dose. Toxic effects apart from intoxication in the early state are mediated by glycolic acid and oxalic acid (metabolites of ethylene glycol). Initially, there is a high osmolar gap due to the presence of ethylene glycol in the circulation.

   Toxic causes of a raised osmolal gap include:
   - Methanol
   - Ethylene glycol
   - Diethylene glycol
   - Isopropanol
   - Ethanol

   As it is metabolized the osmolar gap starts to normalize, but a HAGMA develops due to the formation of glycolic acid and its metabolites, as well as hyperlactatemia [increased NADH (nicotinamide adenine dinucleotide hydrogen) suppresses the conversion of lactate to pyruvate]. Oxalic acid deposits in renal tubules as insoluble calcium oxalate monohydrate, leading to proximal tubular necrosis and renal dysfunction. Oxalic acid's affinity for calcium leads to hypocalcemia, associated with tetany, seizures, and QT interval prolongation.

3. **Discuss the clinical course of severe ethylene glycol toxicity.**
   - *1-2 hours:* State of alcohol intoxication, characterized by euphoria, nystagmus, drowsiness, nausea, and vomiting with high osmolar gap on ABG.
   - *4-12 hours:* Toxic metabolites are formed, high osmolar gap resolves, HAGMA and hypocalcemia occur, with clinical manifestations that include dyspnea, tachypnea, tachycardia, hypertension, shock, coma, tetany, seizures, and death.

- *12-18 hours:* Oliguria followed by acute renal failure and multisystem organ dysfunction including ARDS/cerebral edema and cardiac failure.

    If antidote therapy with fomepizole/ethanol/hemodialysis is not initiated, it can result in coma and death.

4. **What are the investigations useful in a case of ethylene glycol toxicity?**
    - Arterial blood gas analysis—HAGMA
    - Osmolar gap (OG) = (measured serum osmolality) − (calculated osmolarity). A normal osmolar gap is <10.
    - Calculated osmolarity = 2 × [Na] + [glucose] + [urea]
    - Measured osmolarity will include osmolarity contributed by ethanol also.
    - Renal function test and calcium levels—hypocalcemia and impaired renal function are noted.
    - Ethanol levels—in case of coingestion
    - Ethylene glycol levels—not readily available
    - Serum beta-hydroxybutyric acid levels—to rule out alcoholic ketoacidosis as cause of HAGMA.
    - Urine microscopy—look for oxalic acid crystals—pathognomonic for ethylene glycol toxicity.

5. **Discuss management of ethylene glycol toxicity.**

    The goal of management is to inhibit alcohol dehydrogenase enzyme to prevent conversion of ethylene glycol to its toxic metabolites.
    - Assess and support ABC
    - No role of charcoal or gastric lavage as alcohols are rapidly absorbed
    - *Antidote:*
        - *Fomepizole* (4-methylpyruvate)—competitive antagonist of alcohol dehydrogenase:
            - Loading dose of 15 mg/kg
            - Maintenance dosing of 10 mg/kg every 12 hours for four doses, or until the ethylene glycol concentration is at least <62 mg/dL with normal acid-base status.
            - If patient is on dialysis dose needs to be repeated every 4 hours.
        - *Ethanol* also competes with toxic alcohols for conversion by alcohol dehydrogenase. Intravenous administration of ethanol (make 10% ethanol by adding 100 mL of 100% ethanol to 900 mL of 5% dextrose in water):
            - *Loading dose:* 8 mL/kg of 10% ethanol
            - *Maintenance:* 1-2 mL/kg/h of 10% ethanol

    Indications for continued ethanol therapy are:
    - Methanol or ethylene glycol poisoning with blood concentrations[14]
    - >200 mg/L
    - Metabolic acidosis with pH <7.3.
    - Osmolal gap >10 mOsmol/kg water

- Formate concentration >10 mg/L
- Urinary oxalate crystals
- Severe symptoms

Indications for hemodialysis in methanol or ethylene glycol poisoning are:[15]
- Methanol or ethylene glycol concentration >500 mg/L.
- Severe metabolic acidosis (pH < 7.3) unresponsive to therapy, i.e., ABGs are needed in all cases of high-anion gap poisoning.
- Renal failure—hence it is essential to check plasma urea and electrolytes in all patients.
- Presence of visual problems in methanol poisoning.
- Formate concentration >500 mg/L in methanol poisoning.

Hemodialysis should be continued until the methanol/ethylene glycol concentration is <200 mg/L.
- *Progressive coma or respiratory failure:* Intubation and ventilation may be required. A 1 mmol/kg bolus of $NaHCO_3$ prior to intubation may help prevent decompensation due to worsening acidosis. Hyperventilate post intubation to correct the acidosis.
- *Seizures:* Control with IV benzodiazepines, and intubate and ventilate as required.
- *Hypocalcemia:* Correct only in case of refractory seizures or prolonged QT, otherwise calcium administration may contribute to further calcium oxalate crystal formation.
- *Hypoglycemia, hyperkalemia, and hypomagnesemia:* Correct as needed.

CASE SCENARIO 6: METHEMOGLOBINEMIA

A 56-year-old male was admitted to the ER with complaints of chest heaviness. On arrival, oxygen saturation on room air was 87%. He was started on supplemental oxygen at 6 liter with FM. He had history of fever 1 week ago and was taking chloroquine. Chest X-ray and ECG did not reveal any abnormality; cardiac enzymes were within normal limits. Despite O_2 supplementation his saturation levels continues to be 85-87%. His blood sample looks chocolate brown in color and his ABG collected on room air is as follows:

Blood gas values		Reference values
pH	7.42	7.35–7.45
PaO_2 (mm Hg)	97	83–108
$PaCO_2$ (mm Hg)	39.8	32–48
HCO_3^- (mmol/L)	25.3	22–28
Oximetry values		
SO_2 %	96	94–98
FCOHb %	0.3	0–5
FMetHb %	10.3	0–1.5
Electrolyte values		
Sodium (mmol/L)	137	136–145

Contd...

Contd...

Blood gas values		Reference values
Potassium (mmol/L)	3.5	3.4–4.5
Chloride (mmol/L)	104	98–107
Metabolic values		
Creatinine (mg/dL)	2.4	0.45–1.09
Lactate (mmol/L)	1.6	0.45–1.09

1. **What do you infer from the above ABG, and what is the likely diagnosis?**
   His PaO_2 levels are within normal limits with a saturation of 87%. He has elevated methemoglobin (MetHb) levels of 10.3%, indicating methemoglobinemia secondary to consumption of chloroquine.[16]

2. **What is saturation gap and discuss its significance?**
   Oxygen saturation gap is the difference between calculated oxygen saturation from a standard blood gas machine and the reading from a pulse oximeter. If it is >5% there may be abnormal hemoglobin, representing possibility of carbon monoxide, methemoglobinemia, or sulfhemoglobinemia.

   Low SpO_2 readings occur because pulse oximeters utilize light absorption at 660 nm and 940 nm to calculate the ratio of oxyhemoglobin to deoxyhemoglobin in blood. MetHb absorbs light at both these wavelengths; thus, the presence of additional hemoglobin species makes SpO_2 calculations inaccurate.

3. **What are the causes of methemoglobinemia?**
   - Congenital cause—cytochrome 5 reductase deficiency
   - Acquired causes include exposure to drugs such as:
     - Aniline dyes
     - Benzene derivatives
     - Chloroquine, dapsone
     - Prilocaine, benzocaine
     - Metoclopramide
     - Nitrites [nitroglycerine, nitric oxide (NO), sodium nitroprusside]
     - Sulfonamides.

4. **Explain the underlying pathophysiology.**
   Normal hemoglobin contains ferrous iron (Fe^{2+}). MetHb is formed when the ferrous iron in hemoglobin is oxidized to the ferric state (Fe^{3+}). Methemoglobin (Fe^{3+}) is unable to reversibly bind oxygen and it increases the oxygen affinity of any remaining ferrous (Fe^{2+}) hems in the hemoglobin tetramer, resulting in a left shift of the oxygen dissociation curve and reduced O_2 delivery to the tissue.

5. **What are the clinical features of methemoglobinemia?**
   Symptoms are proportional to the fraction of MetHb. A normal MetHb fraction is about 1% (range, 0–3%).[17,18]

- 3-15%—slight discoloration (e.g., pale, gray, and blue) of the skin
- 15-20%—cyanosis, though patients may be relatively asymptomatic
- 25-50%—headache, dyspnea, light-headedness, weakness, confusion, palpitations, and chest pain
- 50-70%—abnormal cardiac rhythms; altered mental status, delirium, seizures, coma; profound acidosis
- >70%—usually death.

6. **How do you manage this patient?**
   - Resuscitation—high flow O_2 (to ensure available Hb is saturated well)
   - Specific therapy includes:
     - Remove from source
     - Methylene blue (1-2 mg/kg over 5 minutes) provides an artificial electron acceptor to facilitate the reduction of MetHb via the NADPH-dependent pathway; give if:
       - Symptomatic
       - Consider if asymptomatic with >20% MetHb, or >10% if risk factors such as anemia or ischemic heart disease
   - Repeat methylene blue at 30-60 minutes if inadequate response:
     - Alternatives to methylene blue:
       - Ascorbic acid [if methylene blue contraindicated, e.g., glucose-6-phosphate dehydrogenase (G6PD) deficiency]
       - Exchange transfusion
       - Hyperbaric oxygen
   - Consider the following if MetHb levels do not fall with methylene blue:
     - Massive ongoing exposure to an oxidizing agent
     - Sulfhemoglobinemia (e.g., dapsone and sulfonamides)
     - G6PD deficiency.

CASE SCENARIO 7: CYANIDE TOXICITY

A 54-year-old male was rescued from fire in a plastic toy manufacturing unit. He was found unresponsive with minimal first degree burns along the upper torso. According to the paramedics he had generalized tonic–clonic convulsions en route to the hospital. Patient had a HR of 128 beats/min and BP of 148/96 mm Hg with saturation of 89% and was started on high flow O_2 with nonrebreathing mask. His initial blood gas analysis is as follows:

Blood gas values		Reference values
pH	7.09	7.35–7.45
PaO_2 (mm Hg)	342	83–108
$PaCO_2$ (mm Hg)	34	32–48
HCO_3^- (mmol/L)	9	22–28

Contd...

Contd...

Blood gas values		Reference values
Oximetry values		
SO_2 %	98	94–98
FCOHb %	2	0–6
FMetHb %	0.5	0–3
Electrolyte values		
Sodium (mmol/L)	137	136–145
Potassium (mmol/L)	3.5	3.4–4.5
Chloride (mmol/L)	99	98–107
Metabolic values		
Creatinine (mg/dL)	1.6	0.45–1.09
Lactate (mmol/L)	19	0.45–1.09

1. **What is the possible diagnosis based on the history and ABG?**

   History of smoke inhalation, unresponsiveness, history of GTCS, and elevated lactate levels with HAGMA without severe burns favors a likely diagnosis of cyanide toxicity. Carbon monoxide poisoning is ruled out based on the COHb levels on the ABG.

2. **Discuss the mechanism of cyanide toxicity.**

   Cyanide exerts its toxic effects mainly by inhibition of cytochrome C oxidase resulting in the following:
   - Binds the ferric (Fe^{3+}) ion of cytochrome C oxidase causing "histotoxic hypoxia" and profound lactic acidosis (as all tissues become dependent on anaerobic metabolism).
   - Results in pulmonary edema and heart failure secondary to release of biogenic amines causing pulmonary and coronary vasoconstriction.
   - Stimulates neurotransmitter release, such as N-methyl-D-aspartate (NMDA), causing neurotoxicity and seizures.

3. **Discuss the clinical features of cyanide toxicity.**
   - Acute inhalation causes rapid loss of consciousness and seizures while oral ingestion causes onset of symptoms in a dose-dependent manner over a duration of 30 minutes.
   - Nonspecific symptoms occur with mild exposures including nausea, vomiting, headache, dyspnea, increased RR, hypertension, tachycardia, altered level of consciousness, and seizures.
   - *Severe exposures:* Associated with end organ dysfunction due to anaerobic respiration and histotoxic hypoxia.
     - Hypotension, bradycardia, reduced GCS and respiratory depression, cardiovascular collapse
     - Hyperlactatemia
     - May appear "pink" due to high SvO_2 following oxygen administration
     - Smell of bitter almonds on breath (not always noted).

4. **What investigations will point toward the diagnosis?**
   - *Blood gas:*
     - Lactate >10 mmol/L:
       - In patients without severe burns, this corresponds to a cyanide level of >40 µmol/L
       - Sensitivity of 87% and a specificity of 94% (positive likelihood ratio of 14.5 and a negative likelihood ratio of 0.14)
     - High SvO_2 with oxygen administration (poor oxygen extraction)
     - COHb (suspect coexistent carbon monoxide poisoning if smoke inhalation)
   - *Cyanide levels correlate with clinical severity:*
     - >20 µmol/L—symptomatic
     - >40 µmol/L—potentially toxic
     - >100 µmol/L—lethal.

5. **What is the line of management for cyanide toxicity?**
   - Remove the victim from the source.
   - Ensure personal safety as cyanide can be absorbed transdermally and by inhalation. Hydrogen cyanide gas is known to be liberated from patient vomitus.
   - Remove any contaminated clothing and wash contaminated skin with soap and water.
   - *Resuscitation:*
     - Avoid mouth-to-mouth/nose ventilation
     - Check ABC:
       - Administer high-flow oxygen, intubation in case of low GCS
       - Provide hemodynamic support:
         - Inotropes/vasopressors
         - Consider extracorporeal support
     - Give antidote if suspected toxicity—hydroxocobalamin then sodium thiosulfate is generally preferred when available.[19]

6. **Describe the role of antidotes in cyanide toxicity.**
   The main cyanide antidotes include:[20]
   - Cobalt-containing cyanide binders—dicobalt edetate and hydroxocobalamin
   - Sulfur donors—sodium thiosulfate, which acts as a sulfur donor to the endogenous rhodanese enzyme
   - Methemoglobin generators—oxidants such as amyl nitrite (inhaled), sodium nitrite (IV), and dimethyl aminophenol (IV/IM).

   Hydroxocobalamin and thiosulfate: These should be administered separately and not together as they form a complex.[21]
   - Administer 5 g hydroxocobalamin diluted in 200 mL of 5% dextrose IV over 30 minutes (binds 100 mg cyanide)—to form cyanocobalamin (Vitamin B_{12}), excreted in the urine.
   - Administer 12.5 g sodium thiosulfate (50 mL of 25% solution) IV over 10 minutes—converts cyanide to thiocyanate—100-fold less toxic than cyanide, excreted in the urine.

Adverse effects:
- *Hydroxocobalamin*—occasional hypertension, bradycardia, or tachycardia (not requiring treatment), orange-red skin and body fluid discoloration (benign, lasts up to 48 hours)
- *Sodium thiosulfate*—nausea and vomiting with rapid injection; minor nonspecific effects such as hypotension, headache, abdominal pain, and confusion.

Dicobalt edetate: It is administered 300 mg IV (7.5 mg/kg in children) over 1 minute followed by 50 mL of 50% glucose.

It can cause seizures, chest pain, hypotension, urticaria, and vomiting. Due to its toxicity, it should only be given in cases of suspected severe poisoning.

Methemoglobin generators: These are contraindicated in the setting of smoke inhalation and possible carbon monoxide poisoning as they are likely to aggravate tissue hypoxia.[22,23]

CASE SCENARIO 8: SALICYLATE TOXICITY

A 75-year-old male was admitted with complaints of difficulty breathing and altered mental status since today morning. He was confused and agitated with tachypnea. Vital signs included a temperature of 36.5°C, BP of 102/83 mm Hg, HR of 105 beats/min, RR of 36 breaths/min, and SpO_2 of 97%. He is otherwise a known hypertensive. He is also diabetic with history of coronary angioplasty done 6 months back. He has been having persistent headaches for the last couple of weeks and has been taking aspirin frequently for the same. His ABG is as follows:

		Reference values
pH	7.54	7.35–7.45
PaO_2 (mm Hg)	76	83–108
$PaCO_2$ (mm Hg)	20	32–48
HCO_3^- (mmol/L)	18	22–28
Base excess	–4	65–95
Lactate (mmol/L)	1.3	0.4–0.8
Sodium (mmol/L)	135	136–145
Potassium (mmol/L)	5.4	3.4–4.5
Chloride (mmol/L)	98	98–107

1. **Describe the mechanism of salicylate toxicity.**

   Ingestion of >150, 250, and 500 mg/kg body weight (BW) of aspirin produces mild, moderate, and severe poisoning, respectively.

   The principle pathophysiologic effects of salicylate toxicity are characterized by:[24]
   - Direct stimulation of the cerebral medulla causes hyperventilation and respiratory alkalosis.
   - Uncoupling of oxidative phosphorylation in the mitochondria. Lactate levels then increase due to the increase in anaerobic metabolism. The lactic acid along with a slight contribution from the salicylate metabolites results in metabolic acidosis.

   Hyperventilation worsens in an attempt to compensate for the metabolic acidosis.

2. **What is the classical triad of salicylate poisoning?**

   The classical triad includes hyperventilation, GI upset, and tinnitus.

   Signs of serious salicylate poisoning include metabolic acidosis, renal failure, and CNS effects, such as agitation, confusion, coma, and convulsions. Death may occur as a result of CNS depression and cardiovascular collapse.

3. **What investigations will point toward the diagnosis of salicylate toxicity?**
   - *Blood gas:* Respiratory center stimulation causes respiratory alkalosis. Uncoupled oxidative phosphorylation and interruption of glucose and fatty acid metabolism by salicylates often causes a concurrent metabolic acidosis.
   - *Salicylate levels:*
     - *Therapeutic range:* 15–30 mg/dL
     - *Mild:* <50 mg/dL
     - *Moderate:* 50–75 mg/dL
     - *Severe:* >75 mg/dL
   - ECG—widened QRS, AV block, and ventricular arrhythmias
   - Hypo-/hyperglycemia
   - Hypokalemia is common.

4. **Outline the management of salicylate toxicity.**[25,26]
   - Assess and support ABC
   - *Fluid resuscitation:* Fluid resuscitate to a goal of 3 cc/kg/h urine output, but be careful to avoid fluid overload.
   - *GI decontamination:* Consider activated charcoal in alert patients with ingestion within 4 hours or massive overdose *after* intubation. Whole bowel irrigation has no role.
   - *Correct electrolyte imbalances before intubation:* Hypokalemia is common.
   - *Intubation:* Give sodium bicarbonate boluses in the periintubation period and maintain a high-minute ventilation by increasing tidal volume and/or RR to keep the serum pH alkalemia.
   - *Match your ventilator to your patient's physiology:* Postintubation aim for high minute ventilation to a goal of $PCO_2 < 20$ mm Hg.
   - *Serum alkalinization is more important than urine alkalinization:* Bicarbonate 1–2 mEq/kg IV bolus, then infusion at 150 mEq in 1 liter D5W maintenance fluid to target serum pH 7.45–7.55.
   - Early hemodialysis for high serum acetylsalicylic acid (ASA) levels (>100 mg/dL), severe CNS effects, pulmonary edema, acute renal failure, and intractable acidosis.

CASE SCENARIO 9: ACETAMINOPHEN TOXICITY

A unresponsive 15-year-old female was brought to the ER. Upon arrival her vital signs are within normal limits other than a mild tachypnea, but she is unresponsive (GCS 5) and is therefore intubated. There are no signs of trauma on her physical examination and a head computed tomography (CT) is negative. She was last seen 6 hours prior after having a fight with her mother. A serum acetaminophen is measured at greater than 800 µg/mL and her serum transaminase activity is normal. A urine pregnancy test and drug screen are negative.

		Reference values
pH	7.254	7.35–7.45
PaO$_2$ (mm Hg)	108	83–108
PaCO$_2$ (mm Hg)	30	32–48
HCO$_3^-$ (mmol/L)	14	22–28
Glucose (mg/dL)	165	65–95
Lactate (mmol/L)	1.0	0.4–0.8
Sodium (mmol/L)	142	136–145
Potassium (mmol/L)	3.6	3.4–4.5
Chloride (mmol/L)	105	98–107
Creatinine (mg/dL)	1.6	0.45–1.09
Lactate (mmol/L)	4.7	0.45–1.09

1. **Interpret the above ABG.**
   Arterial blood gas is suggestive of HAGMA with lactic acidosis in acetaminophen poisoning.[27] It is due to accumulation of 5-oxoproline in patients predisposed to reduced glutathione stores in the early phase or secondary to reduced hepatic clearance, in later stages. But in shocked patients there may also be a contribution of peripheral anaerobic respiration because of tissue hypoperfusion.

2. **What is the toxic dose of acetaminophen?**
   The recommended dose of acetaminophen for adults is 650–1,000 mg every 4–6 hours, not to exceed 4 g/day. In children, the dose is 15 mg/kg every 6 hours, up to 60 mg/kg/day.[28]
   Toxicity develops at 7.5 g/day to 10 g/day or 140 mg/kg.

3. **What are the factors that increase the risk of acetaminophen toxicity?**
   - *Inducers of CYP2E1 (increase metabolism of acetaminophen into toxic NAPQI):*
     - Isoniazid
     - Rifampicin, phenobarbital
     - Phenytoin, phenobarbital
   - *Hepatic depletion of glutathione:*
     - Chronic alcohol ingestion
     - Chronic acetaminophen use
     - Chronic liver disease
     - Malnutrition.

4. **Explain the mechanism of acetaminophen toxicity?**
   Metabolism primarily occurs through glucuronidation and sulfuration, both of which occur in the liver. In an overdose, these pathways are saturated, and more acetaminophen is subsequently metabolized to NAPQI by cytochrome P450.

N-acetyl-*p*-benzoquinone imine is a toxic substance that is safely reduced by glutathione to nontoxic mercaptate and cysteine compounds, which are then renally excreted.

An overdose depletes the stores of glutathione, and once they reach less than 30% of normal, NAPQI levels increase and subsequently bind to hepatic macromolecules causing irreversible hepatic necrosis.

5. **How is acetaminophen toxicity determined?**

   Diagnosis of acetaminophen toxicity is based on serum levels of the drug, even if there are no symptoms.

   If serum levels fall into the toxic range based on the Rumack-Matthew nomogram, then treatment with N-acetyl cysteine should be initiated. A level greater than 150 µg/mL at 4 hours from ingestion is considered toxic. Serum levels must be drawn between 4 and 24 hours from the time of ingestion to use the nomogram properly.

6. **Discuss the stages of acetaminophen toxicity.**
   - First stage (30 minutes to 24 hours)—asymptomatic or may have emesis.
   - Second stage (18 hours to 72 hours)—emesis plus right upper quadrant pain and hypotension.
   - Third stage (72 hours to 96 hours)—liver dysfunction is significant with renal failure, coagulopathies, metabolic acidosis, and encephalopathy. GI symptoms reappear; multiorgan failure and death are the most common at this stage.
   - Fourth stage (4 days to 3 weeks)—patients who survive the third stage are marked by recovery.

7. **How is acetaminophen-induced hepatotoxicity defined?**

   Acetaminophen-induced hepatotoxicity is defined as a peak elevation in hepatic transaminases [alanine transaminase or aspartate transaminase (ALT or AST)] >1,000 IU/L in the context of paracetamol overdose.[29]

8. **Discuss the role of NAC in paracetamol poisoning and the dosing regimen used.**

   The mainstay of treatment for acetaminophen toxicity is acetylcysteine. It replenishes hepatic glutathione stores and increases sulfate conjugation, preventing accumulation of NAPQI. It also improves hemodynamics and oxygen use, decreases cerebral edema, and improves mitochondrial energy production.

   Continuous IV infusion is recommended at loading dose of 150 mg/kg IV over 60 minutes followed by a maintenance dose of 50 mg/kg over 4 hours, followed by a second maintenance dose of 100 mg/kg administered over 16 hours.

9. **Enumerate the criteria to stop NAC after 20 hours.**

   N-acetylcysteine after 20 hours can be stopped if:
   - Acetaminophen concentration is <10 mg/L (66 µmol/L)
   - ALT is <50 U/L
   - International normalized ratio (INR) < 2.0
   - Patient is clinically well.

10. **List the criteria for referral of a patient to transplant unit.**
    - INR > 3.0 at 48 hours or >4.5 at any time
    - Oliguria or creatinine >200 µmol/L
    - Acidosis with pH <7.3 after resuscitation
    - Systolic hypotension with BP <80 mm Hg
    - Hypoglycemia
    - Severe thrombocytopenia
    - Encephalopathy of any degree.

11. **What is the modified King's College Criteria for liver transplantation?**
    The modified King's college criteria are:
    - pH < 7.3 or
    - Arterial lactate concentration >3.5 mmol/L after early resuscitation (4 hours)
    - Lactate > 3.0 mmol/L after fluid resuscitation (12 hours after admission)

    or
    - INR > 6 (PT > 100s) +
    - Creatinine > 300 mmol/L +
    - Grade III or IV encephalopathy.

CASE SCENARIO 10: PARAQUET POISONING

A 34-year-old gentleman was brought to the hospital in a confused state. He allegedly consumed 25–30 mL of 24% paraquat, following a familial dispute 24 hours ago. He was complaining of burning sensation in the mouth, abdominal discomfort, and difficulty swallowing. On examination, there were multiple erosions over his lips and oral cavity, and crepitations in the chest and rest systemic examination was normal. He is started on supplemental oxygen with 2 liter nasal prongs to maintain saturation above 94%. On evaluation, his white blood cell counts were normal, creatinine was 2.12 mg/dL, urea was elevated (97 mg/dL), and he had a hypokalemia with a potassium of 3.1 mmol/L.

1. **Discuss the mechanism of paraquat toxicity.**
   The principal target organ for paraquat poisoning is the lung and kidney. It is actively taken up and concentrates in alveolar type I and II cells due to structural similarity to polyamines. It is also actively secreted by the kidney leading to vacuolation in the cells of the proximal convoluted tubules, thereby causing renal tubular necrosis. Paraquat causes redox cycling and production of toxic reactive oxygen species. This oxidative stress leads to pulmonary damage (alveolitis and fibrosis). Hepatocellular injury occurs secondary to mitochondrial damage and endoplasmic reticulum degranulation.[30]

2. **What are the signs and symptoms of acute paraquat toxicity?**
   Paraquat is a highly toxic herbicide with >50% case fatality rate. The systemic manifestation of paraquat toxicity depends upon the quantity ingested.

   Mild to moderate poisoning—<10 mL of 20% paraquat solution (<20 mg/kg BW): Asymptomatic to mild GI symptoms (nausea, vomiting, and diarrhea) with oral ulceration.

- *Moderate to severe poisoning—10-50 mL of 20% paraquat solution (20-40 mg/kg BW):* Ulceration of mucous membranes (paraquat tongue), renal involvement initially over 2-6 days. Hypoxia after 3-7 days which worsens gradually causing severe hypoxia due to lung fibrosis in 4-6 weeks.
- *Severe to fulminant poisoning—>50 mL of 20% paraquat solution (>40 mg/kg BW):* Esophageal perforation, hypoxia, and cardiovascular collapse with multiorgan involvement. Fulminant course and death ensue in few hours to few days.

3. **What investigations will point toward the diagnosis?**
   - The mainstay of diagnosis is a circumstantial history, evidence of paraquat exposure, and the amount of poison ingested.
   - Sodium dithionite test on urine (if changes color to blue, confirms urine paraquat concentration >1 mg/L, plasma paraquat concentration >2 mg/L) indicates a very poor prognosis)—qualitative assessment
   - Paraquat assay—quantitative assessment
   - Routine complete blood counts, liver function test, and renal function tests must be done. Chest radiographs are also useful in detecting early insult to the lungs (alveolitis), pulmonary fibrosis, acute respiratory distress syndrome, and rarer complications like pneumomediastinum or pneumothorax.
   - Serum amylase and lipase can be done if the patient presents with severe abdominal pain to rule out acute toxin-induced pancreatitis.

4. **Outline the management of paraquat poisoning.**
   - *Airway management and decontamination:*
     - Early nasogastric tube (NGT) insertion is recommended (due to mucosal injury) followed by activated charcoal(1-2 g/kg) or Fullers earth (1-2 g/kg)
     - Avoid gastric lavage as it causes caustic injury.
   - *Ventilation:* Titrate O_2 to target $SpO_2 > 88\%$.
     - Patients requiring mechanical ventilation (MV) usually have a poor prognosis. Early MV may further worsen the fibrosis. Noninvasive or invasive ventilation may be used as a bridge to extracorporeal therapies and lung transplant later.
   - *Hemodialysis and hemofiltration:* Both should be started as early as possible, within 2-4 hours of ingestion, but should be used within 6 hours after that evidence of benefit is very much limited.
   - *Prevention/management of pulmonary fibrosis:*
     - Immune suppression with cyclophosphamide, MESNA (2-mercaptoethane sulfonate), methylprednisolone, and dexamethasone to dampen inflammatory reaction (unproven)
     - Antioxidants such as acetylcysteine and salicylate might be beneficial through free radical scavenging, anti-inflammatory and nuclear factor (NF)-κB inhibitory actions (no evidence).[31,32]
   - *ECMO:* It is used as a bridge to lung transplant. Need for ECMO in the first week of exposure carries grave prognosis.

Toxicology

CASE SCENARIO 11: ALUMINIUM PHOSPHIDE POISONING

A 45-year-old farmer presented with history of ingestion of four tablets of Celphos 4 hours prior to admission. He complains of three to four episodes of vomiting and abdominal pain. On examination, he was agitated and irritable. His HR was 133 beats/min and BP was 70/40 mm Hg. He was tachypneic and pale with a saturation of 91%. His blood counts, renal function tests, liver function tests, and cardiac enzymes were normal. His ABG is as follows:

		Reference values
pH	6.92	7.35–7.45
PaO_2 (mm Hg)	76	83–108
$PaCO_2$ (mm Hg)	17	32–48
HCO_3^- (mmol/L)	5	22–28
Glucose (mg/dL)	165	65–95
Lactate (mmol/L)	13	0.4–0.8
Sodium (mmol/L)	146	136–145
Potassium (mmol/L)	3.4	3.4–4.5
Chloride (mmol/L)	105	98–107

1. **Interpret the above ABG and the underlying mechanism.**

   This ABG is suggestive of HAGMA with very high lactates and very low bicarbonate values. This is a classic example of aluminum phosphide (ALP) poisoning.

   Aluminum phosphide releases phosphine (PH_3) gas as it comes in contact with moisture or air and is rapidly absorbed from gut.[33]

   Phosphine inhibits cellular respiration by inhibition of cytochrome C, preventing cellular respiration, leading to the formation of reactive oxygen species and severe organ dysfunction. The accumulation of lactic acid is because of nonentry of pyruvate into mitochondria. This overwhelms all the alkali reserves and the bicarbonate-generating capacity by the renal system. Thus, all these patients present with HAGMA with very high lactates and very low bicarbonates, with a very low pH (from 6.8 to 7.2).

2. **Enlist the clinical manifestations of ALP poisoning.**
   - *CVS:* Cardiogenic shock with reduced ejection fraction as low as <20%, arrhythmias such as SVT, ventricular tachycardia/ventricular fibrillation, atrial fibrillation, ST-T changes, and conduction defects, especially Bundle of HIS
   - *CNS:* Patients are usually conscious and sensorium is intact initially until hypoxia supervenes resulting in altered mental status
   - *Respiratory support (RS):* Airway irritation, acidotic breathing, foul garlicky rotten fish odor
   - *GI:* Nausea, vomiting, diarrhea, mild transaminitis, and pain abdomen
   - *Renal:* Acute kidney injury and oliguria
   - *Acid–base and electrolytes:* HAGMA, hyperlactatemia, dyselectrolytemia, and hypoglycemia.

3. **How will you diagnose this patient?**
   - Diagnosis usually depends on clinical suspicion or history by patient or attendant.
   - *Odor:* Garlicky or decaying fish odor from the patient.
   - *Silver nitrate test:* Detection of PH_3 gas in exhaled air or in gastric contents. If PH_3 is present then the paper will turn black due to silver phosphate.
   - *Gas chromatography:* It is the most sensitive and specific test to detect even minute amounts of PH_3 in viscera and gastric contents collected during autopsy (mainly used in postmortem)

4. **Discuss the management of patient with ALP poisoning.**
   Due to no known specific antidote, management is primarily supportive care.
   - *Initial assessment and resuscitation:* Circulatory collapse requires immediate attention—intravenous fluids, vasopressor, and inotropic support along with sodium bicarbonate therapy to correct the severe metabolic acidosis are of paramount importance. Early use of IABP and ECMO when indicated have shown favorable outcomes.
     - Fluid resuscitation with crystalloids should be started immediately after measuring central venous pressure or inferior vena cava (IVC) diameter. Large boluses of sodium bicarbonate may be required to correct the severe metabolic acidosis. Frequent ABGs to assess the pH and lactate levels are recommended to maintain a pH above 7.
     - Target Na of 150 mEq/L and blood sugar level of 150–180 mg/dL should be maintained.
     - Vasopressors with invasive arterial BP monitoring to maintain systolic blood pressure (SBP) of 90 mm Hg. Frequent bedside echocardiography is always recommended to monitor cardiac functioning and assess ejection fraction. Persistent tachyarrhythmias may warrant synchronized cardioversion or temporary pacing in case of bradyarrhythmias.
     - Initiate ECMO as soon as possible if patient has severe metabolic acidosis (pH < 7.1), marked LV dysfunction EF < 30%, refractory hypotension SBP < 90 mm Hg even with vasopressor/inotropic support, severe lactic acidosis, lactate > 10 mmol/L), life-threatening arrhythmias, and multiorgan failure.
     - High-flow supplemental oxygen may be initiated to reduce the work of breathing, and positive pressure ventilation when required is an ominous sign as it may further compromise the hemodynamics.
   - *Reduce toxin exposure:* Healthcare personnel should wear proper personal protective equipment (PPE).
     - Decontamination of skin, eye, and other body surfaces as soon as possible to limit PH_3 absorption through the mucocutaneous route.
     - *Gastric lavage:* Useful only if performed early (within 1–2 hours of ingestion).
     - Potassium permanganate (1:10,000) oxidizes PH_3 to nontoxic phosphate.
     - Activated charcoal to reduce absorption if the patient arrives within 1 hour after ingestion of a large amount of poison.

- Vegetable oils and liquid paraffin inhibit PH_3 release from the ingested ALP by coating the stomach with a layer.
- Phosphine excretion can be increased by maintaining adequate renal perfusion and urine output.
  - *Treating metabolic acidosis*: There are three possible methods:
    1. Sodium bicarbonate administration
    2. RRT, HD/sustained low-efficiency dialysis (SLED), results in improvement in pH, LVEF, and BP. Early use of RRT is needed to generate more endogenous bicarbonates during the first 24–48 hours.
    3. Treating the cause and prevent further production of lactic acid.
  - *Other supportive measures include*:
    - *Intravenous magnesium sulfate:* As a membrane-stabilizing agent, free radical scavenger, and antiarrhythmic; needs Mg^{+2} level monitoring.
    - NAC-antioxidant and free radical scavenger
    - Trimetazidine—cardioprotective agent reducing myocardial O_2 consumption
    - *Others:* Glutathione, melatonin, vitamin C, and beta-carotene.

5. **What are the prognostic markers in patients with ALP poisoning?**
   A very low pH <7.0, LVEF <25%, and serum PH_3 levels >1.6 mg/dL are the markers, which correlate with high mortality.

   Arterial pH was cited to be an important prognostic indicator, with very high mortality in those with pH <7.0, hyperglycemia, hyperleukocytosis, and refractory shock with renal failure.[34]

CASE SCENARIO 12: ORGANOPHOSPHORUS POISONING

A 40-year-old male was brought to the emergency department in an unconscious state. There is a strong pungent garlic odor with saliva drooling from the angle of the mouth. His examination revealed HR 49 beats/min, systolic BP of 75 mm Hg, and RR of 35 breaths/min with bilateral crepitations. His GCS is 4/15. Relatives found an empty bottle of chlorpyrifos beside him.

1. **What is your initial diagnosis in this patient, and how do you confirm it?**
   The empty bottle of chlorpyrifos and the clinical presentation of cholinergic toxidrome point toward organophosphorus (OP) poisoning.[35]

   Suppression of cholinesterase activity (butyrylcholinesterase, pseudocholinesterase, or red cell cholinesterase) to less than 25% is evidence of significant poisoning with OP or carbamate compound.

2. **What is the most common presentation of organophosphate compound (OPC) poisoning and underlying mechanism?**
   Organophosphates phosphorylate the serine hydroxyl group of acetylcholinesterase in CNS, MNJ, ANS, and RBC membranes to inactivate the enzyme. Acetylcholine then accumulates within the nervous system and a cholinergic crisis erupts.
   - The dominant clinical features of acute cholinergic toxicity include SLUDGE/BBB—salivation, lacrimation, urination, defecation, gastric emesis, bronchorrhea, bronchospasm, and bradycardia.

- *Features due to overstimulation of nicotinic and muscarinic acetylcholine receptors in the CNS:* Confusion, agitation, coma, and respiratory failure.
- *Features due to overstimulation of nicotinic acetylcholine receptors at the neuromuscular junction:* Muscle weakness, paralysis, and fasciculations.

3. **Discuss the management strategy.**
   Initial resuscitation follows ABC approach:[36]
   - *Airway and breathing:* Airway needs to be kept patent by clearing secretions by suctioning and triple maneuver. Supplemental oxygen should be started if there is evidence of hypoxia. Intubation may be required if there is clinical deterioration. Succinylcholine should be avoided for rapid sequence induction (RSI), since clearance may be delayed due to acetylcholinesterase inhibition by OPC. Nondepolarizing muscle relaxants can be used, but need higher doses.
   - *Circulation:* Rapid fluid resuscitation, rapid atropinization, and use of vasoactive agents for persistent hypotension.

   Administration of atropine should not be delayed for the sake of oxygenation. Simultaneous administration of atropine while managing the airway helps by drying the secretions, clearing the airway, and improving the GCS.

   Atropine is started at an initial dose of 2 mg bolus with doubling of atropine every 2–5 minutes until atropinization (targets for atropinization: HR >100 beats/min, SBP >90 mm Hg, and clear lung fields).

   Gastric lavage should only be attempted in patients who present within 1 hour of ingestion, especially with megadose and only when airway is protected.

4. **What is the role of oxime therapy in OP poisoning?**
   Pralidoxime (2-PAM) and other oximes, such as HI-6 and obidoxime, are cholinesterase-reactivating agents that are effective in treating both muscarinic and nicotinic symptoms.

   The benefit of oxime therapy depends on:
   - *Dose of intoxication:* No role in megadose intoxication as the reactivated enzyme is rapidly reinhabited.
   - Ageing characteristics of the compound—inhibited acetylcholinesterase becomes aged, meaning they cannot be reactivated by oximes. The half-life of aging varies for each pesticide; if dimethyl, the half-life is around 3 hours; if diethyl, the half-life is around 33 hours.
   - Time from ingestion—beneficial when used <6 hours since ingestion.

5. **What is intermediate syndrome and delayed OP coma?**
   Intermediate syndrome is characterized by acute onset of muscle paralysis following the cholinergic crisis or persistence of muscle paralysis after initial muscle weakness during cholinergic phase.
   - Occurs 24–96 hours following acute poisoning.
   - Clinical features include proximal muscle, neck muscle, and respiratory muscle weakness and cranial nerve palsies.
   - Patients require prolonged ventilatory support as the muscle weakness typically lasts 5–7 days but can last up to 1–2 weeks.

Delayed OP coma occurs in patients with severe organophosphate poisoning usually between 4 and 7 days after poisoning.
- The clinical picture often mimic brain death and differentiated from brain death by presence of pin point pupils in delayed OP coma as opposed to fixed dilated pupils in brain death.
- This phenomenon usually lasts 3-5 days and spontaneously resolves.
- It is due to saturation of central receptors by organophosphate compound over time and the delayed presentation is due to redistribution from adipose tissue.

REFERENCES

1. Peter JV, Rogers N, Murty S, Gerace R, Mackay R, Peake SL. An unusual cause of severe metabolic acidosis. Med J Aust. 2006;185(4):223-5.
2. Dempsey GA, Lyall HJ, Corke CF, Scheinkestel CD. Pyroglutamic acidemia: a cause of high anion gap metabolic acidosis. Crit Care Med. 2000;28(6):1803-7.
3. Mizock BA, Mecher C. Pyroglutamic acid and high anion gap: looking through the keyhole? Crit Care Med. 2000;28(6):2140-1.
4. Hedya SA, Avula A, Swoboda HD. Lithium Toxicity. In: StatPearls [Internet]. Treasure Island (FL): StatPearls Publishing; 2022.
5. Adityanjee, Munshi KR, Thampy A. The syndrome of irreversible lithium-effectuated neurotoxicity. Clin Neuropharmacol. 2005;28(1):38-49.
6. Nickson C. (2020). Tricyclic Antidepressant Toxicity CCC. [online] Available from: https://litfl.com/tricyclic-antidepressant-toxicity-ccc [Last accessed August, 2023].
7. Khalid MM, Waseem M. Tricyclic Antidepressant Toxicity. In: StatPearls [Internet]. Treasure Island (FL): StatPearls Publishing; 2022.
8. Kerr GW, McGuffie AC, Wilkie S. Tricyclic antidepressant overdose: a review. Emerg Med J. 2001;18(4):236-41.
9. Ramasubbu B, James D, Scurr A, Sandilands EA. Serum alkalinisation is the cornerstone of treatment for amitriptyline poisoning. BMJ Case Rep. 2016;2016:10.1136/bcr-2016-214685.
10. Fudickar A, Bein B. Propofol infusion syndrome: update of clinical manifestation and pathophysiology. Minerva Anestesiol. 2009;75(5):339-44.
11. Loh N, Nair P. Propofol infusion syndrome. Cont Edu Anaesth Crit Care Pain. 2013;13(6):200-2.
12. Kam PC, Cardone D. Propofol infusion syndrome. Anaesthesia. 2007;62(7):690-701.
13. Iqbal A, Glagola JJ, Nappe TM. Ethylene Glycol Toxicity. In: StatPearls [Internet]. Treasure Island (FL): StatPearls Publishing; 2022.
14. Rietjens SJ, de Lange DW, Meulenbelt J. Ethylene glycol or methanol intoxication: which antidote should be used, fomepizole or ethanol? Neth J Med. 2014;72(2):73-9.
15. Nickson C. (2020). Ethylene glycol inebriation. [online] Available from: https://litfl.com/ethylene-glycol-inebriation [Last accessed August, 2023].
16. Rehman HU. Methemoglobinemia. West J Med. 2001;175(3):193-6.
17. Prchal JT. Clinical features, diagnosis, and treatment of methemoglobinemia. UpToDate. 2018.
18. Nickson C. (2020). Methaemoglobinaemia. [online] Available from: https://litfl.com/methaemoglobinaemia/ [Last accessed August, 2023].
19. Mégarbane B, Delahaye A, Goldgran-Tolédano D, Baud FJ. Antidotal treatment of cyanide poisoning. J Chin Med Assoc. 2003;66:193.
20. Hall AH, Saiers J, Baud F. Which cyanide antidote? Crit Rev Toxicol. 2009;39(7):541-52.
21. Cummings TF. The treatment of cyanide poisoning. Occup Med (Lond). 2004;54(2):82-5.

22. Baud FJ, Barriot P, Toffis V, Riou B, Vicaut E, Lecarpentier Y, et al. Elevated blood cyanide concentrations in victims of smoke inhalation. N Engl J Med. 1991;325(25):1761-6.
23. Nickson C. (2022). Cyanide Poisoning. [online] Available from: https://litfl.com/cyanide-poisoning-ccc [Last accessed August, 2023].
24. Runde TJ, Nappe TM. Salicylates Toxicity. In: StatPearls [Internet]. Treasure Island (FL): StatPearls Publishing; 2022.
25. Helman A. (2017). BCE 64 Salicylate Poisoning. [online] Available from: https://emergencymedicinecases.com/salicylate-poisoning-2/ [Last accessed August, 2023].
26. Long N. (2020). Salicylate toxicity. [online] Available from: https://litfl.com/salicylate-toxicity/ [Last accessed August, 2023].
27. Shah AD, Wood DM, Dargan PI. Understanding lactic acidosis in paracetamol (acetaminophen) poisoning. Br J Clin Pharmacol. 2011;71(1):20-8.
28. Agrawal S, Khazaeni B. Acetaminophen Toxicity. In: StatPearls [Internet]. Treasure Island (FL): StatPearls Publishing; 2022.
29. Nickson C. (2020). Acute Paracetamol Toxicity. [online] Available from: https://litfl.com/acute-paracetamol-toxicity/ [Last accessed August, 2023].
30. Sukumar CA, Shanbhag V, Shastry AB. Paraquat: The Poison Potion. Indian J Crit Care Med. 2019;23(Suppl 4):S263-S266.
31. Gawarammana IB, Buckley NA. Medical management of paraquat ingestion. Br J Clin Pharmacol. 2011;72(5):745-57.
32. Nickson C. (2020). Paraquat Poisoning. [online] Available from: https://litfl.com/paraquat-poisoning/ [Last accessed August, 2023].
33. Gurjar M, Baronia AK, Azim A, Sharma K. Managing aluminum phosphide poisonings. J Emerg Trauma Shock. 2011;4(3):378-84.
34. Mehrpour O, Jafarzadeh M, Abdollahi M. A systematic review of aluminium phosphide poisoning. Arh Hig Rada Toksikol. 2012;63(1):61-73.
35. Holstege CP, Borek HA. Toxiderms. Crit Care Clin. 2012;28(4):479-98.
36. Eddleston M, Buckley NA, Eyer P, Dawson AH. Management of acute organophosphorus pesticide poisoning. Lancet. 2008;371(9612):597-607.

CHAPTER 6

Artifacts

Pramila Chandan, Bindu Mulakavalupil

CASE SCENARIO 1: DILUTED BLOOD SAMPLE

A 72-year-old male, a known case of diabetes on oral hypoglycemic agent (OHA), is brought to the emergency room (ER) with hypoglycemic coma [hemo glucose test (HGT): 40 mg/dL). Neurological status improves after the ER doctor gives him 100 mL 50% dextrose bolus and starts him on infusion of 5% dextrose in view of persistent hypoglycemia. The patient is shifted to intensive care unit (ICU). He is conscious, alert, and hemodynamically stable. The duty nurse collects a venous blood gas (VBG) sample.

Parameters	Values
pH	7.124
PaO_2 (mm Hg)	41
$PaCO_2$ (mm Hg)	47
HCO_3^- (mmol/L)	21
Glucose (mg/dL)	440
Lactate (mmol/L)	1.5
Sodium (mmol/L)	120
Potassium (mmol/L)	2.3
Chloride (mmol/L)	66
Calcium (mmol/L)	0.89

Interpretation

Diluted blood sample

Diluted sample (blood taken from arm with 5% dextrose flowing): Blood sampling contralateral to the insertion site of an intravenous (IV) line is always the first choice. When blood must be drawn proximal to an IV insertion site, dilution and contamination by the infused substance can occur. Each 100 mL of 5% dextrose injection, USP, contains *dextrose, hydrous 5 g in water for injection*. The caloric value is 170 kcal/L. The osmolarity is 252 mOsmol/L, which is slightly hypotonic. The solution pH is 4.3 (3.2–6.5).[1]

Clinical and Laboratory Standards Institute (CLSI) guidelines GP41-Edition 7, also called "Collection of Diagnostic Venous Blood Specimens." The guidelines note that there is a risk of obtaining erroneous and misleading results when drawing blood from a patient with an IV catheter. The guidelines recommend using the opposite arm (not the arm with the IV catheter) whenever possible, and when not possible, collecting the specimen below (distal to) the IV site. CLSI guidelines recommends that the IV be turned off for 2 minutes or longer and that a tourniquet be placed between the IV site and the blood draw site. The guidelines mention that collection above (proximal) to the IV catheter is not recommended and should be done only when all other options for blood collection have been exhausted.[2]

CASE SCENARIO 2: EDTA EFFECT

A painter and decorator aged 43 years, a known case of hypertension, diabetes, and chronic nonoliguric kidney disease, presented with history of malaise, abdominal cramps, nausea, arthralgia, and mild impaired mental status. The physical examination was unremarkable except for abdominal tenderness. Blood investigation—hemoglobin (Hb): 9 g/L; mean corpuscular volume (MCV): 92 fL; white blood cells (WBC): 13,200/mm^3; platelets: 231,000/mm^3; basophilic stippling of erythrocyte noted on peripheral smear; and blood lead levels: 4.18 µmol/L. He was treated initially with disodium EDTA (ethylenediaminetetraacetic acid) 50 mg/kg every 12 hourly for 5 days in view of lead poisoning. On the 6th day, he started complaining of tingling sensation in both upper arms followed by seizures. He was resuscitated and arterial blood gas (ABG) analysis done at that time showed the following results:

Parameters	Values
pH	7.32
PaO$_2$ (mm Hg)	83
PaCO$_2$ (mm Hg)	37
HCO$_3^-$ (mmol/L)	20
Glucose (mg/dL)	88
Lactate (mmol/L)	1.5
Sodium (mmol/L)	132
Potassium (mmol/L)	3.2
Chloride (mmol/L)	103
Calcium (mmol/L)	0.89

Interpretation

EDTA effect

Ethylenediaminetetraacetic acid is a polyprotic acid containing four carboxylic acid groups and two amine groups, with lone-pair electrons that chelate calcium and several other divalent cations including zinc and magnesium. EDTA might interfere with blood sugar control because it can interact with insulin. EDTA can bind with potassium and magnesium and increase the amount of potassium and magnesium that is flushed out in the urine. This might cause potassium and magnesium levels to drop too low.[3]

CASE SCENARIO 3: HEMOLYZED SAMPLE

A 33-year-old female presented with complaints of fever, loose stools, and features of dehydration to emergency department. She was drowsy, arousable, and obeying simple verbal commands. She had—pulse: 110 beats/min sinus tachycardia, blood pressure (BP): 106/58 mm Hg, and oxygen saturation (SpO_2): 98% on radial artery (RA). An ABG sample shows the following results:

Parameters	Values
pH	7.234
PaO_2 (mm Hg)	84
$PaCO_2$ (mm Hg)	47
HCO_3^- (mmol/L)	25.4
Glucose (mg/dL)	100
Lactate (mmol/L)	1.9
Sodium (mmol/L)	140
Potassium (mmol/L)	7.4
Chloride (mmol/L)	113
Calcium (mmol/L)	0.98

Interpretation

Hemolyzed sample

A study done by Lippi et al.[4] showed that the concentration of cell-free hemoglobin increased from <0.5 g/L to 8.9 ± 1.5 g/L in hemolyzed aliquots. In hemolyzed blood, significant decreases were found for pH (−0.2%), PO_2 (−4.9%), SO_2 (−4.9%), COHb (−11%), and Ca^{2+} (−7%), whereas significant increases were observed for PCO_2 (+4.1%), HCO^{3-} (+1.4%), and potassium (+152%).

To prevent hemolysis (which can interfere with many tests):
- Mix tubes with anticoagulant additives gently 4–6 times.
- Avoid drawing blood from a hematoma.
- Avoid drawing the plunger back too forcefully, if using a needle and syringe, or too small a needle, and avoid frothing of the sample.
- Make sure the venipuncture site is dry.
- Avoid a probing, traumatic venipuncture.
- Avoid prolonged tourniquet application or fist clenching, massaging, squeezing, or probing a site.

REFERENCES

1. van Vonderen MG, Voerman BJ, Hensgens BE. Effect of intravenous infusions on laboratory results in blood specimens drawn proximal to the insertion site of an intravenous canula. Neth J Med. 1998;53(5):224-7.
2. Karon B. (2018). Phlebotomy Top Gun: Drawing Blood from a Patient Receiving Intravenous Fluids. [online]. Available from: https://news.mayocliniclabs.com/2018/05/07/phlebotomy-top-gun-drawing-blood-from-a-patient-receiving-intravenous-fluids/ [Last accessed July, 2023].
3. Banfi G, Salvagno GL, Lippi G. The role of ethylenediamine tetraacetic acid (EDTA) as in vitro anticoagulant for diagnostic purposes. Clin Chem Lab Med. 2007;45(5):565-76.
4. Lippi G, Fontana R, Avanzini P, Sandei F, Ippolito L. Influence of spurious hemolysis on blood gas analysis. Clin Chem Lab Med. 2013;51(8):1651-4.

Index

Page numbers followed by *f* refer to figure, *fc* refer to flowchart, and *t* refer to table.

A

Abdominal pain 79
Abdominal tenderness 123
Absolute reticulocyte count 46
Absorption 97
Academia, correction of
    chronic 73
Acetaminophen 113
    toxic dose of 112
Acetaminophen toxicity 111, 113
    mechanism of 112
    risk of 112
    stages of 113
Acetylcysteine 115
Acid-base 116
    balance 1
    disorders 1, 3*t*
    disturbance 96
    status 6, 7
Acidemia 7
Acute coronary syndrome 82
Acute kidney injury 116
Acute paraquat toxicity
    signs of 114
    symptoms of 114
Acute respiratory distress
    syndrome 2
Acute tubular necrosis, polyuric
    phase of 22
Adrenal insufficiency 83, 84
    diagnose 83
Airway
    and breathing 119
    management 115
Albumin 78
    levels affect 30
Albuminuria 66
Alcohol 3, 4, 42
    abuse, chronic 42
    intoxication, state of 103
Aldosterone: renin ratio 85
Aldosterone effect, decreased 27
Aldosteronism
    primary 14
    secondary 14

Alkalemia 6
Alkaline phosphatase
    poisoning 118
Alkalosis, maintenance of 13
Aluminium phosphide poisoning
    116, 117
Alveolitis 114
Amphetamines 95
Anaerobic respiration 108
Anemia 37-39, 44, 64, 69
    aplastic 41
    macrocytic 40, 41
    microcytic 37
    normocytic 43
    pathophysiology of 44
    sideroblastic 39
Aniline dyes 106
Anion gap 96
Antibiotics 57*t*
Anticholinergic effects 100
Anticoagulants, effects of 60
Antidiuretic hormone 83
Antidote 104
    role of 109
Antilymphocyte globulin 56
Arrhythmia 101
Arterial blood gas 1, 22, 64, 83, 90,
    112, 123
Arterial carbon dioxide 2
Artifacts 122
Ascites 69
Asthma 5
Autoimmune hepatitis 79
Azotemia 69, 70
    postrenal 70

B

Bacterial infection 47
Basophil 37
Benzene derivatives 106
Benzocaine 106
Benzodiazepines 95
Bernard-Soulier syndrome 60

Beta-2 agonist 28
Bicarbonate 2, 8, 28, 91
    infusion test 72
    role of 12
Biliary ascariasis 80
Biliary cholangitis, primary 79
Bilirubin 66
Bisphosphonates 33
Blood 66
    count, complete 90
    gas 111
        values 105
    glucose 8
        level 89
    lactate 8
    sample, diluted 122
    tests 39
    urea nitrogen 64, 65
Body, iron status of 39
Bone formation, increased 29
Bone marrow
    aspiration 46
    biopsy 46
    culture 47
    failure syndromes 42
Bradycardia 100, 108, 118
Bronchorrhea 118
Bronchospasm 118
Burns 34

C

Calcium 81
    gluconate 28
    levels 30
Carbohydrate metabolism 8
Carbon dioxide acidosis,
    chronic 13
Cardiac arrest 101
Cardiac arrhythmias 6
Cardiac troponin 82
Cardiovascular collapse 108
Cardiovascular effects 98
Cardiovascular system 6, 34, 100
Catabolic states, extreme 34
Cation exchange resin 28

Cells, redistribution into 34
Central nervous system 5, 34, 52, 100
Cerebral edema 91
Cerebral vasoconstriction 6
Chloride 65, 96
   depletion 13
   responsive alkalosis 13
Chloroquine 106
Cholangitis, primary sclerosing 79
Choledocholithiasis 80
Cholestasis 78, 79t, 80
   evaluate 79
   laboratories 78
Cholestatic pattern 77
Cholesterol components 17
Chronic kidney disease 33
Cinacalcet 33
Coagulation profile 64
Coagulation workup 59
Coma 103
   progressive 105
Conn's syndrome 84, 85
   diagnose 85
   pathophysiology of 85
C-reactive protein 57, 83
   limitations of 58
Creatine phosphokinase 82
Creatinine 65, 72, 96
Cushing's syndrome 14
Cyanide levels correlate 109
Cyanide toxicity 107, 109
   clinical features of 108
   management for 109
   mechanism of 108
Cystatin C 65
Cytochrome C 116

D

Dapsone 106
Dehydration 75
   severe 74
Delta gap 11
Delta method, limitations of 12
Deranged coagulation, case of 59
Dextrose 104, 122
Diabetes 122
   insipidus, nephrogenic 97
Diabetic ketoacidosis 3, 88
   clinical presentation of 89
   diagnose 89
Diarrhea 97, 114

Dicobalt edetate 110
Diethylene glycol 103
Disseminated intravascular coagulation 49, 62, 78
D-lactic acidosis 11
Donor platelets, single 51
Dyselectrolytemia 116
Dyspnea 103

E

Edema 69
Electrocardiogram 75
Electrochemical neutrality, principle of 3
Electrolyte 65, 116
   abnormalities 74, 89
   imbalances
      common 17
      correct 111
   replacement of 90
Elevated aspartate aminotransferase 64
Elevated liver function tests, differential diagnosis on 77
Emergency room 122
Endocrine 29
   effects 98
Endocrinological abnormalities 83
Endoplasmic reticulum degranulation 114
Enterobacteriaceae 66
Enzyme deficiencies, congenital 96
Eosinophil 37
Ethanol 103, 104
   therapy 104
Ethylene glycol 4, 8, 103
   metabolites of 103
   poisoning 103
Ethylene glycol toxicity 104
   management of 104
   mechanism of 103
   severe 103
Ethylenediaminetetraacetic acid 52, 123
Extracorporeal membrane oxygenation, venovenous 52
Extrahepatic cholestasis, causes of 80t
Extrarenal loss 26

F

Familial hypercholesterolemia 17
Familial intrahepatic cholestasis, progressive 79
Fatty acid, reduced 9
Febrile illness 97
Fibrosis 114
Flow cytometry 47
Flucloxacillin 96
Fludrocortisone 73
Fluid
   abnormalities 89
   resuscitation 90, 111
Fluorescence in situ hybridization 47
Folic acid
   level 41
   stores 42
Fomepizole 104
Fresh frozen plasma 61f
Fulminant poisoning, severe to 115
Fungal infection 47

G

Gas chromatography 117
Gastric emesis 118
Gastric lavage 117
Gastrointestinal effects 98
Glomerular excretion, reduced 27
Glomerular filtration rate, reduced 13
Glucocorticoids 83
Gluconeogenesis 83
Glucose 66
Glutathione
   hepatic depletion of 112
   synthetase deficiency 96
Glycolic acid 103
Glycoprotein 60

H

Heart rate 71
Heavy chain disease 18
Hematology analyzer, automated 38
Hemofiltration 115
Hemoglobin
   measurement of 38
   normal 106
Hemoglobinopathy 39

Hemolytic anemia 96
 causes of microangiopathic 48
Hemolytic-uremic syndrome 60
Hemolyzed sample 124
Heparin-induced
  thrombocytopenia
 diagnosis of 53
 differential diagnosis for 52
 risk factors for 52
Heparin-type 52
Hepatitis 79
 B 79
 serology 64
Hepatocellular laboratories 77
Hepatocellular pattern 77
Hepatojugular reflux 69
Hepatotoxicity 113
Histotoxic hypoxia 108
Hydroxocobalamin 109, 110
Hypercalcemia 31-33, 74
 causes of 32
 clinical manifestations of 32
 exacerbate 33
 management of 32
Hyperglycemia 88
Hyperkalemia 27, 69, 75, 76, 105
 clinical manifestation 28
 management 28
Hyperlactatemia 108, 116
Hyperlipidemia 17
Hypernatremia 23, 24, 25*fc*
Hyperosmolar conditions 74
Hyperosmolar hyperglycemic
  state 86
 complications of 88
 management of 87
 signs of severe 86
Hyperphosphatemia 35, 76
 causes of 35
 clinical features of 35
 management of 35
Hypertension 103
Hypertriglyceridemia 17
Hyperuricemia 76
Hypocalcemia 29, 74, 75,
  91-93, 105
 causes of 29
 clinical manifestations of 30
 management of 30
 severe 31
Hypocapnia, effects of 5
Hypochromic anemia, causes of
  microcytic 39

Hypoglycemia 93, 116
 cause of 93
 development of 92
Hypokalemia 25, 26, 74, 76,
  87, 111
 causes 26
 clinical manifestations 26
 management 26
Hypomagnesemia 105
Hyponatremia 19*fc*, 22
 cause of 19, 21
Hypoosmolar hyponatremia
  18, 20
Hypoparathyroidism 29
Hypoperfusion 75
Hypophosphatemia 33, 73, 74
 causes of 33
Hypotension 108
Hypovolemia 75
Hypoxemia 5, 6

I

Illness, chronic 39
Immunoglobulin deposition
  diseases 18
Infection
 diagnosis of 56
 markers 55
 signs of 69
Insulin 28
 deficiency 88
 overdose 92
 secreting tumors 92
 therapy 91
Intensive care unit 52, 122
Intermediate syndrome 119
Intoxication
 chronic 98
 dose of 119
 severe 98
Intra-aortic balloon pump 52
Intrahepatic cholestasis, causes
  of 79
Intrarenal azotemia 70
Intrarenal failure 68*t*
Intravenous immunoglobulin
  therapy 18
Intravenous insulin infusion 91
Intubation 111
Iron deficiency 39
 anemia 39, 44
Isopropanol 103

K

Ketoacidosis
 alcoholic 8
 causes of 9
 diagnose 9
 manage starvation 9
 starvation 3, 8
Ketone 66
 bodies 90
Ketosis 88

L

Lactate 96
 normal value of 9
 production, physiology of 10
Lactic acid, increased 10
Lactic acidosis 3, 8, 9, 11
 causes of 10
Lead poisoning 39
Leukemia, acute 41
Leukocytosis, case of 55
Leukopenia, case of 55
Light chain disease 18
Lipase 81
Lipoprotein X accumulation 17
Lithium 97
 pharmacokinetics of 97
 serial levels of 99
Lithium toxicity 98
 classification of severity of 98
 pathophysiology of 97
 systemic effects of 98
 treatment of 99
Liver disease
 alcoholic 78
 chronic 42
Liver failure
 acute 78
 chronic 78
Liver function test 19, 77, 81
 components of 77
Liver transplantation, criteria
  for 114
Loop diuretics 28, 32
Lymphocyte 37

M

Macrothrombocytopenia 51
Magnesium 9, 65, 90
Mania, acute 98
Mannitol 4

Mean corpuscular hemoglobin 38
Mean corpuscular volume 38
Megaloblastic anemia 41
  absence of 42
  cause of 42
Membrane stabilization 28
Mental retardation 96
Metabolic acidosis 3, 7, 8, 11, 69, 75, 76, 88, 96, 110, 118
Metabolic alkalosis 3, 12, 14
  causes of 13
  compensatory 7
  etiology of 13
Metabolic compensation 6
Metabolic dysfunction 1
Metabolism 97
Methanol 8, 103
Methemoglobin 106
  generators 110
Methemoglobinemia 105
  causes of 106
  clinical features of 106
Methicillin-sensitive *Staphylococcus aureus* 95
Metoclopramide 106
Microangiopathic hemolytic anemia 47
Microcytic hypochromic anemia, causes of 39
Mirizzi syndrome 80
Monoclonal gammopathies, malignant 17
Monocyte 37
Mucous membranes 69
Myalgia 74
Myelodysplastic syndrome 18, 41, 42
Myocardial contractility, decreased 6
Myoglobinuria 74, 76

N

Nausea 103, 114
Nephrotic syndrome 70
Neurologic effects 98
Neutrophil 37
Neutrophilic leukocytosis 56
Next-generation sequencing 47
Nicotinamide adenine dinucleotide hydrogen 103

Nitric oxide 106
Nitrites 106
Nitroglycerine 106
Nonchloride-responsive alkalosis 13
Noninvasive ventilation 33, 95
Novel biomarkers 67

O

Odor 117
Oliguria 116
Oral calcium 31
Oral hypoglycemic agent 122
Oral phosphate binders 36
Organ dysfunction 96
Organophosphate compound 118
Organophosphorus poisoning 118
Osteoblastic activity 29
Oxalate crystals 67
Oxalic acid 103
  affinity 103
Oxime therapy
  benefit of 119
  role of 119
Oxygen saturation 124
Oxygenation, interpretation of 1

P

Pancreatitis 81
  acute 81
  cause of 81
Pancytopenia 45, 46
Paracetamol 96
Paraquat 114
  poisoning 114
  management of 115
  toxicity, mechanism of 114
Parathyroid
  carcinoma 33
  surgery 29
Perl's stain 39
Phenytoin 112
Phosphate 9, 65, 90, 91
  increased 29
Phosphine inhibits cellular respiration 116
Plasma 72
  cell dyscrasia 44
  potassium 72
  renin activity 85

Platelet count 37
  interpretation of 51
Platelet fall, timing of 53
Pneumonia 5
POEMS syndrome 17
Poisoning, moderate to severe 115
Polytrauma, victims of 74
Postobstructive diuresis 73
Potassium 9, 26, 65, 89, 90, 96
  depletion 13
  permanganate 117
  phosphate solution 27
  removal 28
  replacement 26
Precipitates calcium 29
Precipitation factors, treatment of 91
Pregnancy, intrahepatic cholestasis of 79
Prerenal azotemia 70
Prerenal failure 68*t*
Prilocaine 106
Procalcitonin 56, 57
  induction, noninfectious causes of 56
  values 56*t*
Propofol infusion syndrome 101, 102
  developing 102
  management of 102
Prostate, transurethral resection of 19
Prostatic hyperplasia, benign 69
Pseudohyponatremia 17
Pseudohypoparathyroidism 29
Pseudothrombocytopenia 51
Psychogenic polydipsia 20
Pulmonary causes 5
Pulmonary crackles 69
Pulmonary damage 114
Pulmonary edema 5
Pulmonary embolism 5
Pulmonary fibrosis, management of 115
Pyroglutamic acidemia 96
Pyroglutamic acidosis 95, 96
  causes of 96
  risk factors of 96

R

Radial artery 124
Red cell distribution width 38

Refeeding syndrome 34
  risk factors for 34
Renal failure 3, 8, 76, 91
  acute 22
Renal function 64
Renal function tests 65, 89
  urine analysis 65
Renal insufficiency 14, 97
Renal loss 26, 34
Renal toxicity 98
Renal tubular acidosis 71
  types of 72
Renin-angiotensin-aldosterone
    system 14
Respiratory acidosis 3
  acute 7
  chronic 7
  uncompensated 7
Respiratory alkalosis 4-6
  acute 3, 4, 6
  chronic 3, 6
  primary 6
Respiratory dysfunction 1
Respiratory failure 105
Respiratory support 34, 116
Resuscitation 109
Reticulocyte
  count 46
  production index 46
Rhabdomyolysis 74, 75
  complications of 75
  triad of 74
Rifampicin 112
Rotational thromboelastometry
    graph 63f

S

Salicylate 8, 115
  levels 111
  poisoning, triad of 111
Salicylate toxicity 110
  diagnosis of 111
  management of 111
  mechanism of 110
Saline therapy 13
Salivation 118
Saturation gap 106
Seizures 103, 105
Sepsis 10, 34
  diagnosis of 56
  severe 96

Serum
  acetylsalicylic acid, high 111
  alkalinization 111
  electrolytes 89
  haptocorrin levels 42
  homocysteine level 42
  methylmalonic acid 42
  osmolality 68
    calculate 87
    target 87
  potassium 85
  sodium, laboratory assessment
    of 18
Shock 103
  cardiogenic 116
Sickle-cell trait 74
Silver nitrate test 117
Skin tenting 69
Small bowel fistula 4
Smear examination,
    peripheral 51
Sodium 64, 65, 89, 96
  bicarbonate, treatment
    with 101
  nitroprusside 106
  thiosulfate 109, 110
Sorbitol 4
Special coagulation tests 60
Staphylococcus aureus 74
Starvation ketoacidosis,
    pathophysiology of 8
Streptokinase 62
Sulfonamides 106
Sulfonylurea 93
Supplemental oxygen 105
Syndrome of inappropriate
    antidiuretic hormone
    19, 23, 67
Synthetic function tests 78

T

Tachycardia 103
Tachypnea 103
Tetany 103
Thiazide 22
  diuretics 28
Thiosulfate 109
Thrombocytopenia 51-53, 60, 64
  heparin-induced 53
Thrombocytosis 51
Thromboelastogram
    interpretation 61f

Thromboelastography 61f, 63
Thrombosis 53
Thrombotic complications 91
Thrombotic microangiopathy 52
Thyroid 29
  function test 19
Tissue
  hypoperfusion 10
  iron stores 39
  plasminogen activator 62
Total leukocyte count 37
Toxic metabolites 103
Toxicity, mechanism of 100
Toxicology 95
Toxin 8
  exposure, reduce 117
Tranexamic acid 61f
Transcellular shift 26, 27, 28
Transthoracic
    echocardiography 19
Trauma 34
Tricyclic antidepressant toxicity
    99, 101
  management of 101
  mechanism of 100
  systemic effects of 100
  typical of 100
Triglyceride level 81
Troponin 82
  elevation 82
Tuberculosis infection 47
Tubular function, tests of 65
Tubular necrosis, acute 19, 21,
    22, 67

U

Upper gastrointestinal bleed 63
Urea/creatinine ratio 68
Urea, fractional excretion of 68
Uric acid, increased 75
Urinalysis 18
Urinary sodium 67
Urine 68
  alkalinization of 93
  role of 76
  analysis 66, 90
  anion gap 68, 72
  biochemical analysis 67
  biochemistry 68, 70
  causes of green-colored 102
  chloride 68
  collections 66

culture 72
Na 72
osmolality 68
osmolar gap 68
output 73
potassium 68
quantitative measurements in 95
sodium 68
levels, random 73
Urine/serum creatinine ratio 68
Urokinase 62

V

Venous blood gas 25, 27
Ventilation 115
Vigabatrin 96
Viral hepatitis, cholestatic phase of 79
Vital signs 40
Vitamin
 B_{12} 41
 K deficiency 78
Vomiting 13, 97, 114
von Willebrand's disease 60

W

Waldenstrom macroglobulinemia 17
Warfarin 78
Water restriction 20
White blood cell count, interpretation of 55
Whole blood clot lysis index 62

Z

Zoledronic acid 33

EU GSPR Authorised Reprsentative
Logos Europe, 9 rue Nicolas Poussin
1700, La Rochelle, France
Phone: +33 (0) 6 67 93 73 78
E-mail: contact@logoseurope.eu

www.ingramcontent.com/pod-product-compliance
Ingram Content Group UK Ltd.
Pitfield, Milton Keynes, MK11 3LW, UK
UKHW050457150426
5217IPUK00025B/1722